'Ellen Toronto's book demonstrates the acute need for more writings that integrate and examine maternal subjectivity in the field of psychoanalysis. Toronto guides us through the universal issues of recognizing mothers as full subjects and the concrete and theoretical consequences of our failures to do so. Her original analysis of maternal subjectivity as a dissociated self-state that sustains patriarchal structures reveals the depths of the collective trauma that the erasure of mothers' lives entails. Through analytic explorations of myths and cultural history, Toronto unfolds the inherent paradox of the maternal subject and demonstrates the limitations of psychoanalysis and its language-dominant attempts to capture the subject who is impossible to capture, the mother. Although this book is an unapologetic assertion of the maternal perspective, it also offers hope for a future of dismantling the dissociative projections of patriarchy that will allow the mother an existence for herself, for the universal healing of our intersubjective capacities'.

Helena Vissing, *somatic experiencing practitioner and certified perinatal mental health professional*

'*Maternal Subjectivity: A Dissociated Self-State* alerts us to the reality that mothers have been treated as if they were birthing canals with little or no sexual pleasure during the process. In many parts of the world women are still considered their husbands' property. Countless mothers have become depersonalized in many societies and, as a result, become dissociated. They may become so detached that they hurt their children and end up in jail. This volume highlights the need for societies to provide support for mothers before a crisis occurs'.

Daseta Gray, *certified infant/toddler specialist; candidate at The Harlem Family Institute; Sabree Education Services*

'*Maternal Subjectivity: A Dissociated Self-State* continues the much-needed discussion of "Mother" as a subjective presence, one whose existence has long been disregarded as anything other than a womb. Dr. Toronto has included historical, religious, and psychoanalytic perspectives to clarify this absence. She then uniquely makes the case for motherhood as characterized by existential trauma and subsequent dissociation. *Maternal Subjectivity* is a major and original contribution to the psychoanalytic literature; it is a fascinating must-read that integrates history with contemporary thinking and practice. When Dr. Toronto writes about motherhood, your understanding of the lived experience of mothers as more than a womb comes alive'.

Judith Logue, *practicing psychotherapist, as well as supervising, training and teaching psychoanalyst and American Psychological Association life member*

'Interwoven beautifully with personal history and clinical material, Dr. Toronto explores the absence of the maternal subjective from ancient texts to modern day psychoanalytic theory. Her conclusion is striking: that maternal subjectivity is a dissociated self-state. That when we as a culture fail to acknowledge or accept a mother's selfhood, it threatens a woman's ability to "know" herself—the very essence of dissociation. Motherhood, as it currently stands in American society, is where we house or bury internal and relational conflict, our deepest needs and vulnerability, and how Toronto elegantly puts it, "what it means to be fully human". A most timely read for people reexamining the value of motherhood personally and in our society'.

Meredith Darcy, *psychoanalyst, president Section III: Women, Gender and Psychoanalysis, Division (39) of Psychoanalysis of the American Psychological Association*

MATERNAL SUBJECTIVITY

In this book, Ellen Toronto reveals the dissociation of maternal subjectivity from human experience and provides a psychoanalytic exploration of the (non-)history of motherhood to make possible an understanding and appreciation of maternal worlds.

The persistent patriarchal order acknowledges the mother's existence largely as a "womb", a bearer of children, and although her role is essential in the service of the species, we know very little of her story as a person. The absent presence of the mother as an individual subject and collective ignorance about her experiences has constituted an existential trauma, that is, a trauma of non-existence, and it is only by revealing this dissociation, Toronto argues, that we can begin to excavate the stories of individual mothers as they have borne and raised the world's children, and at last realise that the burdens they carry belong to us all.

As a fulsome account of the maternal perspective, which draws from a variety of sources—including historical research, mythological stories and clinical case material—this book will be significant for students of psychoanalysis, feminism and history, as well as psychoanalysts in training and in practice who seek a richer understanding of maternal being.

Ellen L.K. Toronto is an author and psychoanalyst practicing in Spring, Texas. She has published extensively on gender issues and non-verbal communication. She is first editor of *Into the Void: Psychoanalytic Perspectives on a Gender-Free Case* and *A Womb of Her Own*. She and her husband have 4 sons and 11 grandchildren.

MATERNAL SUBJECTIVITY

A Dissociated Self-State

Ellen L.K. Toronto

Routledge
Taylor & Francis Group
LONDON AND NEW YORK

Designed cover image: LUMEZIA © Getty Images

First published 2024
by Routledge
4 Park Square, Milton Park, Abingdon, Oxon OX14 4RN

and by Routledge
605 Third Avenue, New York, NY 10158

Routledge is an imprint of the Taylor & Francis Group, an informa business

British Library Cataloguing-in-Publication Data
A catalogue record for this book is available from the British Library

Library of Congress Cataloging-in-Publication Data
Names: Toronto, Ellen L. K., author.
Title: Maternal subjectivity : a dissociated self state / Ellen L.K. Toronto.
Description: Abingdon, Oxon ; New York, NY : Routledge, 2024. |
Includes bibliographical references and index. |
Identifiers: LCCN 2023006459 (print) | LCCN 2023006460 (ebook) |
ISBN 9781032537955 (hardback) | ISBN 9781032537948 (paperback) |
ISBN 9781003413677 (ebook)
Subjects: LCSH: Motherhood--Psychological aspects. | Mothers--Psychology.
Classification: LCC HQ759 .T723 2024 (print) | LCC HQ759 (ebook) |
DDC 306.874/3--dc23/eng/20230223
LC record available at https://lccn.loc.gov/2023006459
LC ebook record available at https://lccn.loc.gov/2023006460

ISBN: 978-1-032-53795-5 (hbk)
ISBN: 978-1-032-53794-8 (pbk)
ISBN: 978-1-003-41367-7 (ebk)

DOI: 10.4324/9781003413677

Typeset in ITC Galliard
by SPi Technologies India Pvt Ltd (Straive)

In memory of Elizabeth Lynn and Valerie Lynn who died in infancy.
In memory of my mother, Gladys, who mourned their passing.

Contents

Credits List

The author gratefully acknowledges permission to republish the following articles:

Toronto, E.L. (1991). The feminine unconscious and psychoanalytic theory. *Psychoanalytic Psychology*, *8*(4), pp. 415–438, https://doi.org/10.1037/h0079297; used with permission of the American Psychological Association - Journals; permission conveyed through Copyright Clearance Center, Inc.

Toronto, E.L. (1999). The Application of Therapists' Maternal Capacity in Prerepresentational Body-Based Transference and Countertransference. *Psychoanalytic Social Work*, *6*(2); reprinted by permission of the publisher (Taylor & Francis Ltd., http://www.tandfonline.com).

Preface

At the heart of the human experience is the reality that the survival and socialization of the species depends upon those individuals who mother. That person is typically a female but, in any case, it is a person who gives birth, who lactates, who performs the daily minute care of infants including diaper changing, feeding, sleep cycle, playing, bathing, and so on. For middle class mothers it means a continuing round of lessons, homework, dating, hygiene, and the like. For the poor of our society, it involves the possibility of scrounging for food and shelter as an insurmountable daily task. Mother is a presence, absolutely essential for our survival, and yet, collectively, we have failed to recognize her as a subjective being. She is the proverbial "elephant in the room". Her story, her narrative from her perspective, has not been told. She has, for millennia, remained an absent presence; a being beneath whose apron we dare not look. It is this terrain that is the subjective maternal, that I, along with others before me, wish to explore.

Mothers' experience, apart from that devoted to her child, is difficult to encounter because it remains a mystery even to herself. The patriarchal order has not acknowledged her existence except as the bearer of children, male children in particular. Mothers cannot encounter themselves in historical tales, wherein they exist only as desirable objects or essential wombs. We know what they do but we don't document it. We have no record of the daily tedium of childcare. We skirt around the notion of mothering or we call it "instinctual". We do volumes of research about what children need from their mothers. We create lists of requirements in terms of time spent, attunement, containment, as well as a host of behaviors that would challenge any therapist for even an hour. We fail to recognize that this person, this mother, is cooking, cleaning, caring for other children, working at a job, driving kids hither and thither and also attempting to shower occasionally.

As long as this huge allotment of time, and unpaid labor is not examined, it will continue as a mystery, both to the collective and to the mother herself. Mothers will remain outside the corridors of power and will not be able to influence the laws that could make their lives easier. Can we unravel the mysteries of mothering? Can we acknowledge the toil that it takes on individual women? Can we have empathy for their occasional madness? Can we contain within the human story the agony and ecstasy of all that is "mother"? Can we incorporate into our Western society the role of mother, not as "dissociated" but as integral to the fabric of our society, weaving threads of caring into the calcified structure of patriarchy?

I now realize that I began to search for answers to these questions when I was a small child, viewing the world through the lens that my mother provided. She chafed at the restrictions in her life that ostensibly began when she married in 1934. She was a math teacher in our small town of Kenton, Ohio and loved her job. When she married, however, the law required her to give up teaching in case that position might be needed by a man who was the breadwinner. My father was an attorney and we understood that his role was the important one in our family. I watched in despair as my mother grudgingly cooked meals or asked him sweetly for cash. I noted her frustration when he cancelled her credit card and took away her checking account.

I also had begun to realize that my mother was eccentric. She imposed many rules regarding germs of unknown origin. We sometimes bathed twice a day, especially if we had been to dancing class or the swimming pool. Bodily functions were monitored so severely that it seemed that they were not ours but hers to control. The many therapists and analysts that I have had clarified for me that what seemed "normal" was not. My mother became "the mad women in the attic", like the figure of literary fame and the perfect target to blame for my suffering in the offices of therapists.

But as I explored her tragic past in light of what might have been her personal narrative if she could have expressed it, I began to see that the trajectory of her life had been beset with frustration, anger, and heartache. Mom was a sensitive and creative spirit who had been raised by a woman who was something of a tyrant. My grandma was determined that all of her four children would attend the nearby college of Denison University. With limited means it was essential that they qualify for scholarships. It was vital to her goal that homework be perfect. She monitored all of it and threw papers in the fire that were considered below par. She used physical punishment such as a slap or a spanking frequently even for the standards of the day. I believe that my sensitive mother was permanently terrorized.

My mother's terror and angry in her early life were impacted both by my father's indiscretions and yet again by her deep but unprocessed sorrow at the birth of her stillborn baby Elizabeth.My parents had waited long for this child and were understandably heartbroken at her death. For my mother, the wisdom of the day could well have been the empty promise that "she could have more children" though, at her relatively advanced age for childbearing, she would have known that it might not happen.I was not privy to the shame, the guilt, and the anguish she may have felt or the nature of the support system she did or did not have. I am, however, aware that her grief was never processed in her lifetime. At a conscious level she told my older sister and me that Elizabeth would never have done the ornery stuff that we did. Elizabeth would have been perfect. At some point I joined an unconscious pact with my mother in which I would play "dead" and thus replace the baby she had lost. It was only after years of treatment that my wise analyst pointed out that I was enacting that role, playing "dead" so as to assuage my mother's grief.

In parallel circumstances my sister's second child was a baby girl, Valerie Lynn. She died shortly after her birth of Hyaline Membrane Disease which also took the life of Patrick Bouvier Kennedy, the son of John and Jacqueline Kennedy. I was about 16 at the time of the baby's death. As we waited at the hospital I heard my sister's mother-in-law whisper, "She's gone". I was quickly ushered out to the car. Sometime later my sister's brother-in-law came to tell me that the baby had died. It was difficult for him, so I quickly told him that I already knew. I remember little of how the grief was expressed except for the clear memory of my sister's husband weeping at the graveside. It is only now, some 60 years later, that I can access the terrible sorrow I felt. I am astonished that the feelings have remained "underground" for all these years.

I first encountered Betty Friedan and *The Feminine Mystique* in my senior year at college. She wrote of the brilliant women at the Ivy League Colleges who planned to remake the world and who then appeared at the class reunions with a passel of kids and few plans of their own. Those stories began to resonate with me, influenced undoubtedly by the gifted female members of my family who possessed talents that they loved but were never allowed to pursue. I joined the "consciousness-raising" groups of the time where we began to ask questions and contemplate new directions. Over the decades I came to realize the intransigence of patriarchy and the deeply rooted nature of women's prolonged oppression. I watched as rules and laws began to change and new opportunities opened up for women. But as time has gone by, I have also noted that it is single mothers who still live in poverty. It is women who remain the targets of domestic violence, assault, and rape.It is women whose control over their bodies remains at the whim of the government that is in power.

As I have searched and studied I have noted that while progress has occurred in the lives of women, they are still vulnerable to rape the world over. They are consistently paid lower salaries in comparison to their male counterparts; they are largely absent in the roles of presidents, prime ministers, or heads of major corporations. I have considered the solutions—don't go out at night (my mother); get a lot of education but not too much (also my mother); learn martial arts; get married; don't get married. Advice has been given. Men have been encouraged to care. Some do; some don't. But though women's capabilities remain equivalent in the essential tasks of life, they have never achieved parity with men. Patriarchy has prevailed.

What then has been the sticking point? Why has the progress been so slow? I have come to believe that it is at the one place where, at least throughout most of recorded history, males and females differ. It is women who give birth. It is women who, in most circumstances, provide "mothering". If, in some alternate universe, women were not mothers, their progress might have played out differently. That is, women, without the tasks of bearing and nurturing children, could have progressed alongside men. They could have written books, created great art, made scientific discoveries, participated in government and politics. It is mothers, then, whose lives and essential responsibilities, have, by their all-consuming nature, ensured the intransigence of patriarchy.

My thinking has been greatly expanded by those thinkers and theorists such as Gilligan and Snider; Balsam and Rose who have addressed this conundrum. In their book *Why Does Patriarchy Persist?*, Carol Gilligan and Naomi Snider have proposed a very plausible explanation for the intransigence of patriarchy. They state as follows: "Patriarchy steels us against the vulnerability of loving, and, by doing so, becomes a defense against loss" (Gilligan and Snider, 2018, p.9).It is my view that their premise brings us back to "mother" and our first encounter with love and care. Mother stands at the door of life and death; love and loss, and it is her tenderness (or lack thereof) that we cannot contemplate lest we lose it.

Rosemary Balsam in her volume *Women's Bodies in Psychoanalysis* has alerted us to the striking absence of attention or concern regarding the mother's body in psychoanalysis. It is, of course, of great interest to science and medicine but the focus is on the mechanics of the mother's body as it gives birth safely to a healthy infant. The mother's experience of pregnancy or the changes in her body merit little attention.

In *Mothers: An Essay on Love and Cruelty*, Jacqueline Rose greatly amplifies this discussion with her statement that mothers are "the ultimate scapegoat for our personal and political failings, for everything that is wrong with the world, which it becomes the task—unrealizable, of course—of mothers to repair" (Rose, 2018, p.I). The blame that is heaped on mothers in therapy offices is a manifestation of our unwillingness or inability to recognize them as sentient beings. We cannot bear to "know" the burden that they carry for the cruelty of the world.We must maintain a fantasy of "mother" either as an "institution" or an object rather than as a private person.She remains an entity, a womb, a bearer of the species. We continue to politicize her body in our efforts to control both her power and her sorrow.

The burden of guilt from the collective; the centuries of treatment as an object of either derision or idealization; the personal sorrow and loss; and the unrequited tedium of childcare have rendered mother silent, unknown even to herself.Beneath the "joys" she may or may not feel lies her madness; her responsibility without authority; her incessant (and so annoying) worry; her knowledge that if she is not careful her child could die. These are thoughts that she dare not think so she remains a mystery even to herself. As I hope to illustrate, she may become, as did my mother, "the mad woman in the attic"—plagued by a cacophony of voices too terrible to utter.

Like my mother, I was silent for many years. I spoke little except with friends and family. My private world was unknown even to me. I joined the ranks of motherhood with public joy and private terror. With my husband I raised our four sons with all the love and energy that I possessed, shielding them as best I could from the rules and regulations that still resounded in my head. Then after years of analysis I started to find *myself* within the wreckage of my mother's world. But it was only as I began to map out the patterns and pieces of *her* life that I could fully separate. It was as I forgave her that I could become fully myself.

Our mother's world, her privately held experience, has much within it to expand and enrich the human condition. But presently we have only half of her story, that is, the narrative as constructed by patriarchy. If, as Jacqueline Rose has proposed, "we listen to what they have to say— from deep within their bodies and their minds" (Rose, 2018, p.208), we can flesh out the missing part of the human story. We can access the precarious and, yet, strangely fulfilling, experiences of motherhood. We can hear and know the tedium that permeates the daily requirements of caring for the young of our society. We can understand that love does not come cheaply; that it must be replenished; that in a world obsessed with power and acquisition, mothers remain the last bastion of love and care.

Ultimately, of course, this is my journey but it is one that I believe all of us must take. As we seek and "find" our mothers; understand and acknowledge their being; comprehend their love and their sorrow, we expand our own existence for the betterment of all.It is to that end that I dedicate this book.

References

Balsam, R. (2012). *Women's Bodies in Psychoanalysis.* New York and London: Routledge.

Friedan, B. (2001). *The Feminine Mystique.* New York: W.W. Norton and Company.

Gilligan, C. and Snider, N. (2018). *Why Does Patriarchy Persist?* Medford, MA: Polity Press.

Rose, J. (2018). *Mothers: An Essay on Love and Cruelty.* New York: Farrar, Straus and Giroux.

Introduction

Motherhood as defined by patriarchy "defines, constrains, and regulates how women perceive and practice mothering" (Andrea O'Reilly, 2021, p.571). O'Reilly identifies three themes. First—essentialism, in which women are naturally mothers and born with a set of built-in capacities, dispositions, and desires to nurture children; second—mother is to be the central caregiver of her biological children; third—children require full time mothering; fourth—mothers must lavish excessive amounts of time, energy, and money in the rearing of their children.

It is the argument of this book that while the patriarchal structure defines the mother role, it fails to identify her selfhood insofar as it differs from her focus on her children. Highly influential religious texts such as the Old Testament; myths such as the tales of Clytemnestra; and evidence of her "anonymous" contributions in important scientific and cultural discoveries have either failed to acknowledge mother at all or have considered her a commodity, a product, or merely a womb that is essential to the continuation of the male line. The Supreme Court decision of 2022 has solidified this position.

The excision of mothers as persons from our world view is, in my view, systemic. Borrowing from the concept of systemic racism, it is a "theoretical concept and a reality … that is thus embedded in all social institutions, structures and social relations within our society" (Cole,

DOI: 10.4324/9781003413677-1

2020, p.1). The concept notes that Black people were considered as property and were not given a vote. That was, of course, also true of women, who were not given a vote until 1921—within the lifetime of my mother.

The article addresses the systemic and all-encompassing practices and ideologies that give precedence to White people over Black people. The same may be said of the privileging of men over women as enshrined in "each major part of U.S. society—the economy, politics, education, religion" (Cole, 2020, p.2). It is White men who hold "most positions of power [leading to] a serious and well-documented problem of routine discrimination in all areas of life" (Cole, 2020, p.3). Significant aspects of discrimination occur within the family for both women and Black people. Women's labor has been unpaid. (Does that make it slave labor?) Patriarchal religions have, historically at least, named the father as the head of the family with decision-making, discipline, distribution of wealth, and birth rite at his discretion. It is within the family that the role of mother, while absolutely vital, has long remained within the shadows.

Mother remains an absent presence, one that has echoed through the pages of history as a figure that is rarely mentioned and, if she is, not as a person in her own right. She has, I believe, experienced systemic discrimination which, in turn, constitutes "existential trauma", which has been defined by Hoffman as a state of invisibility; of having no discernible presence in a given environment. Mother's place in the world is without definition except as the bearer and caretaker of children.

I will hypothesize that if mothers were studied as intensely as infants, the results would show that their internal world would bear the signs of trauma to some degree. That is, the mothering experience, precious as we all hope that it is, would in reality contain many hardships. Mothers cannot describe what it feels like to be a mother in the idealized version to which we may subscribe. They might produce a "greeting card" definition but it would bear little resemblance to their inner reality. While their outer reality might be portrayed as joyful and utterly fulfilling, their inner experience may be beset with hardship and even trauma; cultural, physical, familial, and private. That hidden world would, I will argue, constitutes a dissociated self-state.

As Hoffman has stated, existential trauma threatens the very nature of existence. Under that broad heading, I will endeavor to identify societal, religious, governmental, and individual forces that have greatly minimized or even erased the maternal narrative from our collective reality. Their trauma resides in our unconscious as a phenomenon that has saturated the culture. The stories, often glorified, of rape and incest have become a part of our collective view of women and mothers. To illustrate my point I have chosen examples of mothers from myth and religion. They are well-known stories that have become part of our current culture—reference points or perhaps justifications for the way in which women who are mothers are currently treated. The well-known tale of Clytemnestra has been the focus of studies by Rose, Jacobs, and Stone in that she experiences both the inhumane treatment of mothers as well as the circumstances in which they cannot protect their own children. The women of the Old Testament experience similar dealings as victims of rape and incest. They exist primarily in their function as a womb and are, in fact, referred to as such. Otherwise, their presence is rarely mentioned at all. They are tangential to the ongoing story.

The individual experiences of childbirth and childcare may, from some perspectives, also be considered traumatic. Since women's bodies bare almost no mention in traditional psychoanalysis, their experiences as females or child-bearers do not merit mention as being traumatic. Relational psychoanalysis considers the importance of the mother-infant bond but only from the perspective of the infant's needs. While theorists have apparently uncovered the optimal situation for the child—that is, engagement, mirroring, and the like—the difficulties in providing that "facilitating environment" are not considered. For example, the intergenerational trauma that a woman has known would greatly impact her ability to respond to her infant. The non-verbal nature of the baby's communication is addressed but the mother's challenge in finding within herself that long-ago nonverbal language is not.

In their book *Why Does Patriarchy Persist?*, Gilligan and Snider contend that the structure of patriarchy, based in dominance and acquisition, requires a detachment from feeling, and love. Nowhere is this conflict more evident than in a collective determination to erase mother, that is, mother as subject, from existence. Her role as caregiver is fraught with vulnerability, suffering, and loss. If we do not acknowledge her presence and her voice, we have no need to provide a balance between the structure that has made losses irreparable and the need for love that has rendered them inevitable.

Mother as object, not subject, has long served the tenets of patriarchy, that is, a gender binary; the dominance of men over women; and the admonition that men may have "selves" while women must be selfless—serving the needs of men and children. Mothers must be chaste so that the patrilineal bloodlines remain pure. The combined silence of men and women about women has ensured the continuance of patriarchy over millennia in such a way that it has become mistaken for nature. Motherhood as it personifies the vulnerability that accompanies loving, caring, and the commensurate and inevitable losses that occur is perceived as a weakness that threatens the prevailing order. The nature and expression of feelings are perceived as a danger to the demands of power and wealth. The human need to engage becomes an unspoken casualty.

The scales have never yet been balanced, either historically or presently. Mother in her consummate role as the ultimate earthly source of human vulnerability and love has remained in the shadows, idealized or denigrated but never fully known. She is an image, a statue, a concept of mythic proportions even as she stands at the portals of life and death. Babies die. Fetuses perish within her womb. As John Donne has spoken, "We have a winding sheet in our mother's womb" (Donne, 1632). As the initiator of life, she also brings us into mortality where we will inevitably die. She carries the agony of loss, not as a redemptive and holy experience—the Pieta—but as drowning sorrow that is passed on through generations.

Mothers meet us in our infancy, that is, our state of greatest dependence and vulnerability. They bear us and they preserve our lives when we cannot. We typically rely on them throughout our childhoods. The images of mothers and children fleeing Ukraine, or the manner in which pandemic mothering was gendered, expanded, and continually devalued (O'Reilly, 2021, p.916), have confirmed yet again their vital role. O'Reilly cites a study that reports that before the pandemic, men spent an average of 33 hours of caregiving weekly while women spent 68 hours. After the pandemic, men spent an average of 46 hours, and women, 95 hours. Women who mother are not unlike the first responders and healthcare workers who were initially lauded but finally and continually overwhelmed by the onslaught of the sick and the dying.

Jacqueline Rose states that mothers are "the ultimate scapegoat for our personal and political failings, for everything that is wrong with the world, which it becomes the task—unrealizable, of course—of mothers to repair" (Rose, 2018, P.I). To this I would add that it is her role both as the arbiter of life and death and as the ultimate caregiver, that is, the one who bears us and turns us into human beings, that cannot be recognized. Mother personifies both our guilt and our vulnerability. We must maintain a fantasy of "mother" either as an "institution" or an object rather than as a private person and a sentient being whose subjectivity we can acknowledge. She thus remains an entity, a womb, a bearer of the species. We continue to politicize her body in our efforts to control her awesome power.

Following Rose, it is the unformulated "mind of mother" wherein the experiences of love and vulnerability are sequestered and contained. But because she is invisible even to herself, her transcendent joy, unbearable grief, and her awareness of the horrors that we inflict on one another, remain unprocessed and, yes, inflicted upon her offspring. It is only as we recognize mother as an individual, a full participant with her own subjective experience in the human equation, that we can understand and ameliorate her madness to the ultimate benefit of all who know her.

In approaching this conundrum I will, like Jacqueline Rose, endeavor "to travel the world and cross epochs—from South Africa to Ancient Greece; from present-day America to slavery and its legacies … Framing the whole project has been the anguish of mothers and the hostility unleashed against them" (Rose, 2018, pp. 90–91). In the Old Testament she is a womb—significant only as the bearer of sons. In myth she is Clytemnestra—a pawn of the brutal Agamemnon as she watches him cut their daughter's throat before her eyes. In traditional psychoanalysis she is the inferior of the species, caught up in her desire for the phallus. In relational psychoanalysis, she is, sadly enough, an environment—significant to the life and progression of the child—but without attention either to her thoughts as they pertain to the child or to her own deliberations that have little or nothing to do with "him".

The argument will endeavor to find the "real" mother within her place in the patriarchal culture; the psychoanalytic definition that considers her only from the perspective of the child; her necessary immersion in the nonverbal world of the infant. The benevolence of men will not bring her out of the shadows. Patriarchy will not voluntarily give up its power. Rather, it is mother herself who must find her voice. Psychoanalysts excel at giving their patients a voice. We can and we must address ourselves to that issue, that is, finding the voice of *mother as herself* in whatever form it may appear. We can then bring mother out of the shadows, balance the grip of patriarchy, come to terms with our own narcissism, and illuminate the fragile and yet loving existence of "mother".

The structure of the book follows the words of Andre Green who has stated:

> When an analyst assembles a number of … papers into a book … the collection reveals that ideas which seem to be developing in a new way … had already been germinating many years before. Of course the idea when first formulated existed only in a rudimentary form.
>
> (Green, 2018, p.16)

Borrowing from Green, I will begin with my own early articles that reflect the female experience as it differs from patriarchal mandates.

References

Balsam, R. (2012). *Women's Bodies in Psychoanalysis*. New York and London: Routledge.

Bollas, C. (2017). *The Shadow of the Object: Psychoanalysis of the Unthought Known*. New York: Columbia University Press.

Cole, N.L. (2020). *Definition of Systemic Racism in Sociology*. https://www.thoughtco.com/systemic-racism-3026565. Accessed 21 July 2020.

Donne, J. (1632). Sermon given at St. Paul's Cathedral. London, England.

Gilligan, C. and Snider, N. (2018). *Why Does Patriarchy Persist?* Medford, MA: Polity Press.

Green, A. (2018). *On Private Madness*. New York: Routledge.

Hoffman, L. (2013, August). Existential Issues in Trauma: Implications for Assessment and Treatment. *Conference: 121st Annual Convention of the American Psychological Association*. Honolulu, HI.

Jacobs, A. (2007). *On Matricide*. New York: Columbia University Press.

O'Reilly, A. (Ed.). (2021). *Maternal Theory Essential Readings*. Bradford, Ontario: Demeter Press.

Rose, J. (2018). *Mothers: An Essay on Love and Cruelty*. New York: Farrar, Straus, and Giroux.

Stern, D. (2003). *Unformulated Experience*. New York: Psychology Press.

Stone, A. (2012). *Feminism, Psychoanalysis and Maternal Subjectivity*. New York and London: Routledge.

Chapter One
"The Feminine Unconscious"

This chapter began my professional quest of the "mystery" that is mother. It assumes a gender binary which reflects my awareness at that time. I had observed the over-weaning presence of patriarchy as the theoretical groundwork of my psychoanalytic institute and of many of my colleagues, both male and female. I had become increasingly aware of the ways in which that perspective constrained the female experience both in practice and in the male-biased way in which data about women was even collected. Simone de Beauvoir describes women as being in the service of the species while man defines its history. Unlike lower animals however, woman is self-conscious and capable of abstract thought, autonomy and self reflection and thus experiences a painful contradiction.

The article presupposes a primary feminine experience, that is, one that does not borrow from patriarchy and the primacy of the phallus. It addresses the conflict that women face between the needs of the species and those of the individual. It does not as yet consider the semiotic versus the symbolic or the need to "kill" the mother of infancy. Yet it highlights the problem of data collection in that women's experience, particularly as mothers, is sensory-bound—difficult to capture in the guise of language.

DOI: 10.4324/9781003413677-2

It further assumes, however, a gender binary of cis-gender males and females. It does not address the fluidity of gender which confounds, of course, the primacy of patriarchy. Nor does it consider the gender possibilities within the task of mothering. It characterizes mothering as that nurturing role that consists of caring for infants and children in the time-consuming, arduous days and years of unacknowledged labor that "mothering" requires. It assumes that women have done and still do perform the great bulk of mothering and that they do so in unacknowledged recognition and silence. I continue to hold that view.

The case study describes a divorced woman in her forties from a family of five siblings. In the beginning of treatment she was virtually unable to put her feelings into words. She could not describe her emotions while, at the same time, feeling those emotions. As I have stated, her father was something of a tyrant—policing both words and thoughts within the family. The mother was described as being extremely passive and virtually silent—speaking only on rare occasions. My patient refused to enter the patriarchal world in which her father was a skewed example. Her silence was an effective (and maddening) resistance but was, at the same time, paralyzing for adequate functioning in the world.

We may also speculate, given the theories of Kristeva, Irigaray, and Lacan, that she was attempting to remain in her mother's silent universe. She refused to leave and thus "kill" the mother of her infancy. She, in this way, resisted the oppression of patriarchy represented by her father and also kept hidden the madness of her mother and herself.

The article follows.

A primary feminine experience is presupposed. Our collective resistance to knowledge about such an experience is seen as arising out of a patriarchal world view which defines man as subject and woman either as maternal object of the child or sexual object of the man. The article addresses the impact of patriarchy and, particularly, male sexual aggression on the developing female. The problems of collecting data about the feminine unconscious, given the male bias of our theories, are also discussed. Finally, early and modern theories about the primary feminine experience are presented along with illustrative clinical material. Emphasis is placed on woman's reproductive and relational capabilities as well as on her development as a sexual individual, arising out of early and ongoing vaginal awareness.

Psychoanalytic theory has ascribed to the human male a powerful developmental force carrying him from infancy through various stages of psycho-sexual development resulting in an end point of maturity as male.

He emerges as the dominant figure of the species fully capable of possessing at least a reasonable facsimile of his original love object. Traditionally, however, we have perceived no such certain path for the female. Rather we have described a tortuous and uncertain route in which she must first give up her mother, then her longings to be a man, and then at long last find her femininity only when it is benevolently given to her by a man.

Why, as so many have asked, is the path to womanhood, the search for femininity, so uncertain, so shrouded in mystery? How does the human female, presumably existing passively and in the shadow of the male, actively ensure her own survival? If we postulate a feminine unconscious, a primary experience which is from start to finish female, of course intermingling with the male but neither defined nor limited by his needs, are we still faced with many puzzling questions? What form would such data take? What would be its symbols, its metaphors? Would they appear in modalities other than language? Why do we have abundant data from clinical material as well as myth, literature, religion, and art which suggest otherwise, that is, that the woman's longing is indeed exclusively toward the male as has been traditionally proposed?

I concur with many who in recent years have postulated a primary feminine experience, to appearances ephemeral, fleeting, contradictory, but in reality, vibrant, powerful, and purposeful. To ascertain such an experience we must first acknowledge the complex biological and cultural environment which has not only blinded us to the realities of the female experience but also distorted women's actual experiences of themselves as they have attempted to function in a male-dominated world.

In order to understand fully the impact which this complex environment has had upon the development of women we must be fully cognizant of the pervasiveness of maleness. It is now a widely held contention that the outer world, in the official version anyway, was invented by men. As originally and perhaps most eloquently described by Simone de Beauvoir (1949/1952), man is the subject, woman is the Other. Man is the narrator. He is telling the story, explaining the world from his point of view. We are familiar with Horney's assertion that "our whole civilization is a masculine civilization. The state, the laws, morality, religion, and the sciences, are the creation of men" (Westcott, 1986, p.1).

How did this state of affairs originate? How did man come to be the narrator of the human story? Again de Beauvoir (1949/1952) described a complex interweaving of ontological, economic, social, and psychological factors emerging out of the data of biology and the vastly different roles which men and women play in the creation and preservation of the species. It is these differing roles which ensure that man will emerge as the individual whereas woman, even though at the highest level of animal life, will remain to a large extent embedded within the species. De Beauvoir pointed out that, as we go up the scale of animal life, individuality is more and more highly developed. She stated:

> In the mammals, life assumes the most complex forms, and individualization is most advanced and specific. There the division of the two vital components— maintenance and creation—is realized definitively in the separation of the sexes... The female organism is wholly adapted for and subservient to maternity while sexual initiative is the prerogative of the male. ... The female is the victim of the species.
>
> (de Beauvoir, 1949/1952, pp.22–23)

The inherent conflict between the interests of the individual and the interests of the species assumes its most profound and agonizing form in the human female. Like the human male and apart from the female of any other species, she is fully cognizant both of her existence and her autonomy. Yet like the female of all lower life forms she remains wrapped up in the species which literally resides within her and absorbs much of her individual life. Thus it is de Beauvoir's assertion, and one with which I concur, that it is the male's role and position as the most fully developed individual which has given him the vantage point from which to tell the human story in its current patriarchal form.

Our current world view then is male. We have been led to assume that it presents men's and women's subjective experience with equal clarity. I believe however, that this viewpoint might be more accurately described as a mirror, one which confirms and idealizes the male experience and defines women only insofar as they substantiate that experience. Woman's story exists on the dark side of the mirror. Finding their needs, priorities, values, and experiences ill-fitting in a masculine world, women have formed a sort of counter-culture, passed down over the centuries by word of mouth, in personal diaries and journals, in myths and nursery rhymes, in secret and often unconscious ways from mother to child and, more specifically, from mother to daughter. Only in recent times has there been any public recognition of a legitimate feminine world view which differs, often markedly, from the prevailing masculine one.

The task before us then is a difficult one as we seek to discover woman's story despite a complex of factors which obscure our view. Her impressive role in the preservation of the species ensures that her story will be profoundly relational. As such, it is a healthy and positive adaptation to the human condition, one which males could profitably emulate. Insofar as woman's investment in the care of the young has been considered a biological given, the relational aspect of her development has been paradoxically both assumed and, until recently, largely ignored. Yet this relational component in itself already represents a compromise, an accommodation to the heavy demands of species survival. For like the male she, too, is also an individual caught up in what Freud tells us are "a good part of the struggles of mankind …round the single task of finding an expedient accommodation—one, that is, that will bring happiness—between this claim of the individual and the cultural claims of the group" (1930, p.96).

Yet she is uniquely human, possessed of autonomy, will, initiative, aggression, and sexual desire, developing, I argue, out of an early and ongoing awareness of herself as a sexual individual, albeit in a context of significant relationships. Like the human male and apart from the female of any other species, she is fully cognizant both of her existence and her autonomy. Yet like the female of al lower life forms she remains wrapped up in the species which literally resides within her and absorbs much of her individual life. Thus it is de Beauvoir's assertion, and one with which I concur, that it is the male's role and position as the most fully developed individual which has given him the vantage point from which to tell the human story in its current patriarchal form.

The conflict of the individual against civilization is felt at once by both male and female. As de Beauvoir wrote: "In the species capable of high individual development, the urge of the male toward autonomy which in lower animals is his ruin—is crowned with success" (1949/1952, p.27).

It is the woman whose individuality is at risk. It is her story as individual subject which is difficult to extricate both from the shadow of the male and from her existence always "in-relation". Yet she is uniquely human, possessed of autonomy, will, initiative, aggression, and sexual desire, developing, I argue, out of an early and ongoing awareness of herself as a sexual individual, albeit in a context of significant relationships.

How then do we ascertain the experience of the woman as individual? I wish to consider this question from three different angles. First, I consider the consequences of male dominance and the threat of male sexual aggression for the development of women I believe that in many ways the psycho-sexual development of women under patriarchy has been that of a people both oppressed and under siege. As I thought of clinical examples which would illustrate this point, I came to the realization that I could not think of any female patient for whom sexual threat or sexual domination were not a significant aspect of her experience. Secondly, I examine the ways in which our very methods of data collection, possessing in themselves a male bias, have made it difficult to ascertain the primary feminine experience. Finally, I consider some hypotheses about the primary feminine experience. I focus on those theories which postulate a primary feminine experience involving both a conscious awareness of reproductive and relational capabilities and a primary cathexis of female genital organs.

THE PATRIARCHAL MYTH

The male world view with its assumptions of male dominance, the primacy of the phallus, and the law of the Father is at present the prevailing myth of the human social order, relating men to women, mothers and fathers to daughters and sons. It takes the two classes of people in the world—men and women—and orders them: men first, women second. Buttressed as it is by biological factors, religious doctrine, and centuries of tradition, it has the force of an edict, a postulate, a universal truth. It is a myth for both men and women but an extremely powerful one. It captures for all of us the ascendance and triumph of the human male. He has seemingly defeated the forces of nature and is master of all he surveys. He has achieved autonomy, individuality, and the belief that he alone is in control of his own destiny.

Woman, on the other hand, is one of the forces of nature and, as such, a constant reminder of human frailty, mortality, and insignificance. She must be subjugated and in fact participates in her own subjugation. According to French psychoanalyst Lacan (Mitchell, 1984), the feminine then comes to stand for the frailty and vulnerability of the human condition. We can repudiate this subordinate class as missing, incomplete, castrated, feminine. Whether male or not, we can comfort ourselves with the notion that at least some of us are complete and invincible. The concept of woman with an independent, subjective, feminine experience of her own presents another, often precarious, view of the theory of male dominance, independence, and invincibility.

More than a cultural phenomenon, the patriarchal myth draws heavily on the data of biology, emphasizing both real anatomical differences and the vastly differing roles which men and women play in reproduction.

It is highly plausible then that concepts such as penis envy and female inferiority become part of the psychological reality of both boys and girls. Mitchell stated: "To Freud if psychoanalysis is phallo-centric, it is because the human social order that it perceives refracted through the individual human subject is patrocentric" (1984, p.274).

His theory provides a perfect description of women under patriarchy. It is Mitchell's thesis, and one with which I concur, that the tenets of this theory have been translated at deep unconscious levels and thus have become part of the reality of the development of individual women. Women experience themselves as being inferior because they have been taught that they are so at cultural, familial, and individual levels over many centuries. Traditional theories of female psycho-sexual development accurately depict the development of an oppressed class.

The patriarchal myth places man, that is, the human male, at the center of the universe. Created in the image of a male God, all human and animal life revolves around him and exists for his pleasure. Conflicts traditionally center around the transfer of wealth, power, and love objects from one generation of males to the next. Freud told us that it is to the individual's advantage to learn to work in groups and families which will join together to protect his interests. Yet it is man's role as individual—father, leader—which is to be envied and protected and from which he derives the most pleasure (Freud, 1930). The penis itself becomes the ultimate symbol of his power as an individual. As conceivably the greatest source of energy known either to primitive or modern man, at least as an individual, the penis comes to represent the elemental power of the individual male. It is his to use and control at his own discretion, initiative, and pleasure. Of course the limitations and prohibitions surrounding its use are formidable and, arguably, represent the central conflict of psychoanalysis. Yet once he has negotiated the cultural sanctions surrounding his sexuality it is his to own and control as the embodiment of individual pleasure and power. The penis as the representation of such privilege becomes an enviable organ indeed.

Stoller (1975) suggested that without some recognition of the primacy of the phallus symbolically portrayed throughout history in myth, folktale, artistic production, and religious worship, we fail to acknowledge a significant cultural influence on sexual development. Individual sexuality as symbolized by the penis is male. Indeed, the psycho-sexual stage of genital awareness and discovery is named for the male organ. When questioned as to why this convention applies, an experienced male analyst answered, "There's no other name for it". Roheim (1945) presented material which suggests that men unconsciously assume that only men can have orgasms. In order, then, for a woman to achieve orgasm she must either possess a phallus or become a man. Libido itself is viewed as essentially masculine. The impact of this symbolism on the development of both girls and boys is as yet undetermined but undoubtedly significant.

The myth of patriarchy and the theory which describes it presents us with a seemingly orderly universe. All of us have agreed that males are dominant and that the phallus, a universal symbol of sexual privilege, is their unique possession. The law of the father exists to keep their power in check. With the father as the possessor of the phallus, keeper of the law, and protector of his property, that is, his women, we are presumably protected from male sexual aggression and its impact on the sexual development of women. Supporting a kind of patriarchal narcissism, we come to believe that all activity originates from the male and though women may suffer at the hands of men, it surely must be suffering that they enjoy as part of their subordinate status. If we can hypothesize that women enjoy pain and domination, if we can theorize that female patients' reports of rape, incest, and sexual exploitation by their father, are exclusively wish fulfillment and fantasy, then we need not be concerned with the very real suffering of the Other, that is, women.

Horney's descriptions, however (Westcott, 1986), reveal quite a different picture of female sexual development, one in which women experience real suffering and real danger from male sexual aggression. Her evidence reveals an almost routine, though not explicitly incestuous, sexualization of girls, defining them as essentially sexual beings and treating them in seductive and sexually suggestive ways. Her data show households not under the influence of patriarchal authority and renunciation of impulse, but rather as a setting for male sexual conquest, an "emotional hothouse". Fathers and sons are essentially male colleagues and competitors in pursuit of family women. Females are unprotected by the father's power or his internalized authority in the consciences of his sons. The father's right to conquest is the problem itself. Westcott suggested (1986) that the very common occurrence of female sexualization and exercise of male power blinded Freud to the real danger which women fear. If Freud had seriously considered the family landscape of sexualization, he would have implicated the behavior of all men, including himself.

The myth of patriarchy and its many manifestations in clinical data then represent a significant portion of the psychic reality of both men and women. To summarily dismiss such a theory is to dismiss a substantial portion of women's experience and the fact of their oppression.

I believe that this point is illustrated by two sessions with a woman in her forties from a family of five siblings. She is a divorced woman who has had difficulty supporting herself, even though she is intelligent and holds a college degree. In a session she stated that even though she was poor and unimportant she wanted everyone to know how rich, successful, and important her father was. Though not always delineated so directly, this has been a theme throughout her treatment. One could take this as admission of her own inferiority and her implacable envy of her father and his power. Such an interpretation would not account for the patient's own growing awareness of the illusory nature of this power and the terrible price this illusion has extracted from members of the family. I approached it from the point of view that her investment in her father's wealth and power was in fact a barrier to her own ability to formulate career plans and provide for herself. At the next session the patient appeared dejected, disheartened, as though she had suffered some narcissistic blow. She stated that she was unloved and misunderstood by everyone, including me. After some exploration I made the interpretation that my failure to acknowledge her father's power and importance for its own sake had been a grave insult to her. Her mood and manner brightened immediately as we discussed how significant her father's importance was to her own sense of well-being. Thus, although the patient herself recognizes much of the falseness and destructive-ness of this power, it is nevertheless an important aspect of her own grandiose self which must be acknowledged and worked through.

At one level of psychic reality we have, then, as Tenbusch (1987) stated, "patriarchal construction of women which has in turn created our sense of who we are" (p.3). It is a significant aspect of women's psycho-sexual development which cannot be dismissed. It becomes limiting, prejudicial, and, in my opinion, morally reprehensible when it is employed to perpetuate existing biases and when it is assumed to represent the totality of women's experience, despite considerable evidence to the contrary. It does not represent the full and total experience of being a woman. Though little girls may genuinely envy the potential and power of men just as little boys may envy and desire that of women, much of the theory in which females' so-called envy of the male is far greater than the reverse describes the response of an oppressed class to the desires and demands of its oppressors. Therapies bogged down. Interminable analyses. Eroticized transferences. How many of these represent failed attempts to encapsulate the totality of women's experiences within a theory which describes only a part?

PROBLEMS OF DATA COLLECTION

Traditional theory describes the male-dominated culture and experience, just as Newtonian physics describes the physical universe. Understanding the feminine unconscious requires a leap to hyper-space where different conditions, different methods of data collection, and different phenomena prevail. Once again it is the male's vantage point as the quintessential individual of the human species which has profoundly influenced both the form and content of our shared data about the human psyche. Man as the theorist for both sexes has created a world which places him at the center of interpersonal and familial relationships. Male psycho-sexual development has traditionally been the standard by which all individual development has been interpreted. Indeed, theorizing itself may be seen as a male activity, "a victory of intellectuality over sensuality" (Freud, 1939, p.114), particularly when it involves the breaking down of human experience into discrete, analyzable bits of data. Male-dominated thinking has failed to acknowledge feminine thinking which is heavily relational, contextual and sensory bound. In order then to bring the data of the feminine unconscious into the mainstream of human thought, we as therapists must first acknowledge that the theories through which we hear, understand, organize, and interpret data are in themselves male-centered and male-biased ways of cognizing experience.

The relative importance of the theory in the mind of the therapist may vary. Yet it is highly unlikely that as therapists we ever operate without a theory of some sort, one which undoubtedly reflects our biases about the relative places of men and women. At one extreme, all data are organized to fit the theory and the therapist's understanding of the data is then conveyed to the patient. Almost any response by the patient is presumed to represent confirmation of the interpretation. Data which do not fit the theory are misperceived or ignored. An example of this approach is described by Brenner (1976) in which a female patient's fear of flying and particularly her inability to control the situation while flying were attributed to her inability to have and control the "joystick", that is, penis, which is used to control an airplane. Though it was unclear from the description, this connection appears to have been based on Brenner's associations rather than the patient's. Brenner stated, "If one knows what the controls of an aircraft look like … for this patient to sit at the controls unconsciously gratified her wish to have a penis herself" (1976, p.151). It has been pointed out to me, however, that airplanes have not had joysticks since before World War II. In this instance, neither data from the patient nor data from external reality appears to have had a bearing on the validity of the interpretation. Other approaches determine the meaning of data only in the context of the new history being created between patient and therapist (Leavy, 1985). Harris pointed out, however, that analytic discourse is rarely democratic and that "one must particularly address the question of what set of interests or entitlement allows interpretation … [an] innocent query can mask control and direction" (1985, p.23). Even the Oedipus complex, broadly defined as "unconscious representations of parent-child interactions" (Leavy, 1985, p.5), already presupposes some sort of family structure which has traditionally placed women in subordinate positions. There is in no way a symmetrical balance of power between men and women. The father is the universal arbiter of the law; the mother, the object of desire. The feminist version of the oedipal crisis reads as "the familial moment in a general social system in which women are exchanged" (Harris, 1985, p.22). Yet with few exceptions this is a central concept around which data is organized.

Other examples of the heavy male bias in traditional theory are provided in Kulish's (1990) paper on the mental representation of the clitoris. Kulish noted Freud's consistent bias in his view of the clitoris as a substitute penis. This is apparent in his description of the clitoris as a penis that "remains permanently stunted" (Freud, 1909, p.12), as well as in his view that the clitoris is represented in the dreams of women as a phallus (Freud, 1917). Kulish further pointed out that Freud continually transferred his own experience of male sexuality onto women and girls. This is manifest in his belief that sexual excitement in women occurs in the form of "spasms" (Freud, 1905, p.220) or thrusts, just as it does in men. It is Kulish's view, as well as that of Kestenberg (1975) and Montgrain (1983), that women's experience of sexual excitement is circular rather than linear in nature. Women's experience of genital anxiety, which according to Glover and Mendell (1982) is most frequently felt and expressed as penetration anxiety, is all too often misinterpreted as symbolic of castration anxiety (i.e., fear that the penis has been or will be removed). Contributing to the male bias in traditional theory is the fact pointed out by Lerner (1976) that female genital parts are frequently either mislabeled or ignored. Perhaps the most glaring and obvious male bias in the psychoanalytic account of female sexual development is the belief which Freud (1905, 1931, 1933) expressed that the vagina is unknown both to little boys and little girls. This view has proved remarkably intransigent over the years despite considerable theoretical, clinical, and scientific data to the contrary. Such a viewpoint is, I believe, the result of massive cultural and individual repression of woman's sexuality on many fronts. Our adherence to this belief, however, and our organization of data around it, leaves women without a sense of ownership of their own sexuality. Forever sexual objects, both to themselves and to men, they are denied the sense of competence, personal causation, and self-affirmation which sexual subjectivity brings.

It is the point of view of Lacan that the male bias within our culture is embodied within language itself. Thus, in his view, as soon as we attain language we enter a system of signifiers in which the words masculine and feminine already carry weighty definitions (Mitchell, 1975). Language is viewed as a linear, goal-oriented mode, representative of the symbolic, the superior, the law of the father. The structure, that is, language, clearly delineates the relationship between men and women, with the phallus being the essential signifier of the relationship between the "haves" and the "have-nots". The father, whether present in reality or not, is the possessor of the phallus and the embodiment of the privileged group. It is the father via the threat of castration who arbitrates the relationship between mother and child and puts the lid on incestuous wishes. Thus the female enters language alienated and objectified, already in submission to the law. The Lacanian position is, in my view, an extreme one. Yet it does point out the pervasiveness of patriarchal assumptions. It is also unquestionable in my mind that language and culture are deeply intertwined, the one being an accurate and veridical reflection of the other. Schafer (1973) addressed this point in what he called "the problem of naming" (p.477). He stated:

> To designate is also to create and enforce. By devising and allocating words, which are names, people create entities and modes of experience and enforce specific modes of experience. Names render events, situations, and relationships available or unavailable for psychological life that might otherwise remain cognitively indeterminate.

Schafer is referring specifically to Freud's equation of feminine with passive submissive, and masochistic and masculine with active, dominant, and aggressive. He suggested that Freud may have originally been "simply naming" (p.478) that is, devising verbal conventions. But for Freud, as for the rest of us, names become edicts, moral prescriptions, and statements of the essential differences between men and women. Language comes to dictate culture and vice versa. The close fit between the two has profound influence on psychological reality and the expression of that reality. The data of the analytic situation are predominantly, if not exclusively, linguistic. Hence they already possess a heavy masculine bias.

To summarize, traditional psychoanalytic theory, like the preponderance of Western thought, has placed man at the center. The male body is viewed as the standard model, and man as the subject around which familial and interpersonal relationships revolve. Even language and abstract thought are viewed as masculine, a "turning from the mother to the father" (Freud, 1939, p.114). To the extent that all of us are human, this theory has provided rich data about the feminine unconscious. Yet there is a strong and growing awareness that much about the feminine experience has been ignored, unrecognized, misperceived, and lost. Traditional theories simply don't fit the data. In order to recapture this data or perhaps discover it for the first time, we must re-orient our thinking around those theories which, for the time being at least, place woman at the center. Such an apparently radical premise brings into focus immediately a number of assumptions which traditional theory has either minimized or failed to acknowledge.

First of all, any theory which attempts to comprehend fully the feminine experience must acknowledge that women are relational. They exist in a continuing state of relatedness. Jordan (1989) stated that Western science, including psychology, is based on an assumption of a primary reality composed of separate objects which secondarily come into relationship with one another. Moving from Aristotelian logic and Newtonian Physics to quantum physics, we begin to see reality defined by relationships, continuities, and probabilities rather than by discrete objects and dualities (p.1). Such innovative assumptions of course call into question the traditional view of the male as the primary individual as well as his alleged independence, security, and separateness from other people.

A second assumption, critical to woman-centered theories, is that women are and probably always will be sensory bound. Furthermore, sense perception is a mode of knowing which, contrary to Freud's view, is not necessarily inferior to thought perception or intellectuality. Our heavy reliance on language and rational thought is limiting for both sexes, but particularly so for women, for whom the strikingly nonverbal world of the infant is so salient. To be mothers, women must be and are trained to rely on nonverbal cues. Their so-called intuition undoubtedly partakes heavily of these factors. The "tyranny of language" excludes a significant portion of feminine modes of perceiving and experiencing the world around them. Indeed, it is Goldstein's viewpoint (1984) that it is men, alienated from the mother-child matrix, who have substituted intellectuality and abstract thought for the knowledge of the senses. Acknowledging the feminine experience mandates that we open up avenues of data collection relying on smell, touch, and other nonverbal modalities. Though the ultimate goal of psychoanalysis may be the transformation of the unconscious into symbolic (i.e., verbal) form, it is extremely limiting to assume that it would only be encoded and expressed as language at all points along the way.

Thirdly, our development of woman-centered theories must acknowledge that although women may possess heightened sensory capabilities, they are also fully capable of abstract thought. Intellectuality is not a masculine prerogative. Mitchell warned (1984) that the world of the presymbolic, the intuitive, and the mysterious is the domain to which women have already been relegated under patriarchy. We must not be seduced into believing that exploring the feminine side forever plunges us into the abyss, the silent, the unknowable. It might appear so, but it must not remain so. Kaplan (1983) stated that women must not remain outside the historical process. They can and must find a voice, learning to speak from the void, "creating a kind of underground, a sort of rupture through negativity" (p.93). The challenge is to face the unknowable and render it known, to probe the mysterious and learn its symbols, its patterns, its laws.

The final point which I believe feminist theory must address is the recognition of woman as subject. She is neither a pale imitation of the masculine nor wholly defined in relation to others. She is herself—an individual. She possesses a primary feminine nature and experience, defined in part at least through her feminine body. She develops in and through her body, which is profoundly different from the male body and which cannot be understood through male experience and metaphor. Her sexual development, though at risk in relation to the larger and more aggressive male, has a course and impetus of its own. Woman is relational and individual, symbolic and sensory. She possesses all of these characteristics, contradictory only when any are denied. Like wave and particle theories of light, all are accurate characterizations under appropriate conditions and circumstances.

A clinical example of the tyranny of language and the need for alternative methods of data collection is provided in the treatment of the divorced woman referred to earlier. Her family of origin could be described as a caricature patriarchy. Her father seemingly wielded absolute power and demanded total obedience, not just of action but of feelings and will. She described situations in which her father would demand that toys be put away. If the task was not done exactly as he desired he would physically force the child to pick up the toy in exactly the way he desired. My patient described having her hands forced into the dishwater by him as an adult so that she would wash dishes appropriately. The patient's mother appeared rigidly passive and avoided any and all situations wherein there would be any suggestion of a separate identity for her. She was depressed and rarely spoke at all. It was regarded as an event in the family when the mother actually talked.

After many years of treatment, it is still extremely difficult for this woman to put her feelings into words. It is not possible, for example, for her to say she is sad while feeling sad. Blandness and lack of affect are striking, as well as vagueness of verbal descriptions and responses. I was extremely puzzled by this and for a long time thought it to be a passive stubbornness and resistance on her part. I have since come to view it as alexithymia (a condition usually brought on by extreme early trauma in which feeling and cognition must be separated by massive repression). I believe that for this woman to accede to the symbolic world of words and language would be to capitulate totally to the oppression which she experienced and further to a sense of her own nothingness. She is caught between the symbolic world of her father, wherein she was defined as non-existent, and the silent world to which her mother withdrew.

Even a seemingly innocuous question such as "Can you tell me what you are thinking?" is experienced by her as a command much like her father would give. She is still far from being able to put her inner world into words. Only as we have been able to understand this difficulty has she been able to move forward. I have frequently made the interpretation that for her to talk at all is already to be co-opted into a system and set of rules which she did not invent. To remain silent is also dangerous but it allows her to retain some sense of control and freedom. She has, however, progressed to the point that she can describe certain bodily sensations or somatic memories which occur in reaction to something she is talking about. She will say, for example, that her whole body feels "tense" or that her legs feel "heavy". I believe that these experiences represent extremely important data not as yet available in verbal form.

In spite of her difficulties with language, this patient has thus managed to communicate in nonverbal sensory modalities. Changes in posture, body language, and manner of dress have provided striking evidence of her increased self-esteem over the course of treatment. Early in treatment another notable feature was that when she appeared distressed, often before or after my vacation, a peculiar odor emanated from her. It was not associated with lack of cleanliness but was sharp and acrid in quality. It was in fact never verbalized by either of us but nevertheless contributed to my understanding of her. She and I have slowly come to understand her world through the realization that words do not always mean what we think they mean, that language can be a barrier as well as a bridge, and that silence is sometimes not resistance but survival. Our goal will not of course be to leave this woman without the access which verbal expression provides. But the attainment of the goal will be a recognition that data are data in whatever form they take and that words, when they come to her, will be her words, an expression of her uniquely feminine self.

THE PRIMARY FEMININE EXPERIENCE

The patriarchal myth is just that, a myth for both men and women. As such it elucidates only part of human experience and is thus limiting for both sexes. Until recently, our acknowledgment of the other half of human experience has been spotty, fragmentary, a glimpse here and a glimpse there. Phenomena such as hysteria, witchcraft, silence itself, have provided tears in the cloak of patriarchy, but the totality of feminine experience has not been acknowledged as a legitimate world view able to explain a vast wealth of data. We are finally discovering, however, that beneath the supposed bedrock of penis envy and masculine protest flows a vibrant, bubbling underground spring of primary feminine experience.

An encompassing theory of such an experience must acknowledge not only woman's reproductive and relational capabilities, but also her uniquely human growth as an individual. From her viewpoint as an experiencing subject, we can comprehend her deep involvement in the reproduction and nurturing of the species, not as a mere pawn of biological destiny, but as an active participant who understands and values her role as life-giver and caregiver and who decides how and when she will participate in this aspect of her life. We can also understand her development as a sexual being with accompanying desires for self-affirmation, personal causation, and competence.

Psychoanalytic feminism has in recent years defined with great clarity the relational capabilities of women. Qualities of affiliativeness, relatedness, empathy, and nurturance, all of which are largely dismissed or devalued in a male-dominated culture, have been reclaimed and brought into individual and group consciousness. As Jordan (1989) pointed out, these formulations necessitate a re-evaluation of the concept of self as a discrete entity. For both men and women it is separateness, not connectedness, that needs explaining. In *Feminism and Psychoanalytic Theory*, Chodorow (1989) distinguished two strands of psychoanalytic feminism which emphasize the development of healthy adult women in a continuing state of relatedness and attachment. The object relations school, drawing heavily from Chodorow's own work, *The Reproduction of Mothering* (1978), focuses on the mother-daughter relationship. Chodorow (1989) stated:

> Through their early relationship with their mother, women develop a sense of self continuous with others and a richly constructed, bisexual, oedipal oscillating with pre-oedipal inner self-object world that continuously engages unconscious and conscious activity: The basic feminine sense of self is connected to the world.
>
> (p.184)

The interpersonal group, heavily influenced by Miller (1976) and Gilligan (1982), also stresses the development of women's "self-in-relation". Though there are some important distinctions between the two schools of thought, both approaches call into question the often-stated goals of independence and autonomy as the acme of adult mental health. When we acknowledge in a conscious and directed way the significance of women's relational capabilities, we are faced with a far less certain concept of the mentally healthy individual. Our psychological reality is at all moments male and female, oedipal and pre-oedipal, certain and uncertain, product and process, separate and connected, analytic and intuitive, verbal and visceral, knowable and unknowable. Furthermore, as Schafer (1973) pointed out, this necessitates a re-evaluation of the crisis of the oedipal stage which emphasizes the "cutting of" of pre-oedipal ties with the mother.

Schafer stated:

> … to be consistent with psychoanalytic propositions and findings, one must see the girl and later, the woman as being in a profoundly influential, continuously intense and active relationship, not only with her real mother, but with the idea and imagined presence of her mother …
>
> (p.476)

The ultimate ideal of heterosexual pairing as the goal of adult development implies a separateness, a relinquishing of other relationships for this exclusive pairing. It also involves the notion of competition and conquest, particularly for the male, and the ideal of exclusivity, particularly for the female. This presupposes independence and autonomy for each individual partner and a merging of boundaries only in this exclusive love relationship. There is much to suggest that this presupposition is not accurate for women. Their capacity for relatedness becomes a liability, however, only when it is denied and denigrated as archaic or borderline. Given full recognition and understanding, it becomes an integrative explanatory concept.

Traditional psychoanalysis has, of course, differed from object relational theories in its emphasis on development as mediated through body zones and on the sexual object choice of the individual. The ego has been conceptualized as a "body ego"—a male body ego. In recent years, however, writers such as Chasseguet-Smirgel (1976) and Kestenberg (1968, 1982) suggested that the development of the female, cognized through her feminine body and with a growing awareness of her role in reproduction, is profoundly different from that of the male. Just as interpersonal theorists emphasize woman's relational self as central, recent psychoanalytic writers stress that her reproductive capabilities are in fact a central organizing aspect of her psychosexual development. Such a view differs in important ways from the patriarchal view of motherhood either as biological destiny or as a means of finally gaining the approval and recognition which women seek from the male. It is a view which emphasizes that woman's reproductive capability is not a substitute for thwarted masculinity but is instead, from the beginning of her life, primary in her psychosexual development. Furthermore, that capability need not be understood as a terrible hardship imposed upon her as some passive cog in a great evolutionary machine. It is rather an awesome creative power which is hers to partake in, often joyfully, as an individual experiencing subject. Women, as well as other females in the animal kingdom, share a vital and central role in the preservation of the species. Yet unlike other females, women alone have the capacity to cognize and comprehend their godlike power. It is a power which they, as individuals, literally hold over life itself. It is little wonder, then, that men in their drive toward ascendancy have attempted to institutionalize this power and wrest it from the control of individual women. As Jungian analyst Neumann stated:

> It is the adolescent ego that is still so uncertain of itself that it perceives the female as threatening... an adult male ego [is] one which is able to enter into a creative connection with the Great Mother ... both in her dark and her benign aspects since full adulthood requires eventually entering into some creative relationship with death itself.
>
> (Neumann cited in Rich, 1976, p.118)

Early writers such as C. Thompson (1969) and Fromm-Reichmann and Gunst (1969) discussed the ancient, unconscious psychological devaluation of female sexuality and creativity. Fromm-Reichmann and Gunst stated:

> ... if men are frightened by and devaluate this capacity of women, there is only one way for women to gain appreciation from and be protected by men. They must do this by first concealing from men their genuine pleasure in their natural creativity. Then ... they must conceal their pleasure from themselves and lay stress upon the other side of their roles: the pain of labor ... the discomfort accompanying pregnancy and ... menstruation.
>
> (p.77)

Fromm-Reichmann and Gunst went on to state that, if we define neurosis as the barring of sexual fulfillment and the barring from awareness of sexual satisfaction, then we have created in women a culturally induced neurosis by barring from their awareness the gratifying and sexually satisfying act of procreation. Deutsch and Benedek (1969) have maintained that parturition is the culmination of the sex act for women. Benedek (1960) maintained that whereas for men sexual pleasure begins and ends with coitus, for women, it is a two-stage process. It begins with the orgiastic experience and ends with parturition. A women's sexual life is not circumscribed by the physiology of orgasm but by a complex organization of a woman's personality which enables her to fulfill her function in the reproduction of the species. Benedek went on to describe in a compelling way the outward goal-directed heterosexual tendencies (intended to bring about copulation) fused with a self-directed receptive tendency (designed to facilitate conception), and the parallel of these outward and inward tendencies with the ovarian cycle. This is not to imply that a woman is at the mercy of her hormones as the widely held myth suggests, but that her reproductive capabilities are a highly significant aspect of her biological and psychological life. As with any other area of life, it becomes threatening, irrational, and out of control only when it is repressed, ignored, or denied. Its derivatives must be understood and placed within the conscious awareness of individual women, therein becoming an integrative rather than a disruptive force in the totality of their development.

More recent authors have indeed suggested that the female reproductive capability, the capacity to nurture within one's own body another human life, associated as it is with complex hormonal factors, is in fact translated into the psychic reality of the developing female. It is an enormous power and one which must engender desire, envy, fear, and pleasure just as does male sexual potency, also inaccessible to the growing child. Chasseguet-Smirgel (1976), in accord with Kestenberg (1968), suggested that from the beginning, babies have an idea and a wish for procreation and identification with the mother. She argued that in some way babies understand the idea of the interiority of the mother and the idea of a vagina. According to Chasseguet-Smirgel (1976), the archaic matrix of the Oedipus complex consists of the infant's fantasied wish to return to or rediscover a smooth universe, without obstacles—the mother's womb—and get rid of the father and his penis, which represent the barriers to the mother's womb. Kestenberg (1968) stressed the female preoccupation with inner spaces. Barnett (1966) suggested that the complete sequence of normal female development may be based totally on orifice and cavity cathexis—the lips and mouth, anus and rectum, introitus and vagina.

The female maternal capacity is central to our understanding of the feminine unconscious particularly if we recognize that there are two distinct aspects to mothering. One is the biological act of giving birth and the other, the complex and highly socialized, non-instinctual nurturing capabilities which enable women to care for and raise children. But Freud (1933) himself reminded us that woman is also an individual:

> But do not forget that I have only been describing women insofar as their nature is determined by their sexual, i.e. reproductive function …we do not overlook the fact that an individual woman may be a human being in other respects as well.
>
> (p.135)

It is, I believe, this aspect of woman as individual, an actively experiencing sexual subject, which is most difficult to extricate from her role either as maternal object of the child or as sexual object of the male.

One of the tenets of psychoanalytic theory is that it is critical to the developing ego to gain awareness of oneself as a sexual being. As P.Thompson (1977) pointed out, concepts such as competence, ego strength, mastery, and effectance, all of which relate to a sense of personal control of our own lives, arise out of our growing sexual awareness. The Lacanian position is that subjectivity emerges out of unconscious sexual drives (Chodorow, 1989). Yet the traditional viewpoint has held that female sexuality, apart from the reproductive aspect, is largely a passive, borrowed experience. Individual sexuality has been conceptualized primarily as male. However, a growing number of psychoanalytic writers, beginning with early dissidents such as Jones (1927) and Horney (1933), have argued for the concept of primary femininity, a primary cathexis of female genital organs.

The concept of vaginal awareness is highly significant in our understanding of female development. Parenthetically, I might add that whenever this particular topic is raised, I have invariably observed intense discussion, heated argumentation, and vociferous denial which have led me as a clinician to conclude that this is a very important topic as well as a source of anxiety for many. One might well conclude with Kestenberg (1968) that the universal repudiation of femininity is based on the anxiety-provoking nature of inner genital sensations. There is not, however, a dearth of clinical data around this issue. Numerous writers such as Chasseguet-Smirgel (1976), Kestenberg (1968, 1982), Fraiberg (1972), Greenacre (1950), Wrye (1983), Kramer (1954), Chehrazi (1986), Montgrain (1983), Kleeman (1976), Glover and Mendell (1982), and others have presented clinical data which suggest early vaginal awareness. In addition to clinical data, the data from Masters and Johnson's (1966) laboratories provide further support for the notion of early vaginal awareness. They found that vaginal and clitoral orgasms are indistinguishable physiologically and that vaginal responsiveness always accompanies clitoral stimulation and vice versa. It is extraordinary that this data has, however, been dismissed out of hand as having no bearing on the psycho-sexual development of girls or boys. Eissler (1977), for example, reiterated Freud (1933), who stated "there are a few isolated reports of early vaginal sensations, but it could not be easy to distinguish them from sensations in the anus or vestibulum; in any case they cannot play a great part..." (p.118).

The clinical data relating to vaginal awareness at least in the patient population frequently take the form of unbearable and overwhelming excitement and a resulting flight from the genitals which as Fraiberg pointed out (1972) results in a genital anesthesia in childhood and is the prototype for frigidity in later years. Horney (1933) cited fear of rape and penetration, dread of the male penis, and anxiety about injury to the inside of the body couched in numerous metaphors such as "criminals who break through windows or doors, men with guns who threaten to shoot … animals or women stabbed with knives; animals which creep, fly, or run inside some place (e.g., snakes, mice, moths)" (p.64). Other references reflect anxiety about the injurious consequences of masturbation, such as the following: "crossing a bridge which suddenly breaks off in the middle … walking along a slippery incline which all at once begins to slide … in danger of falling over a precipice" (p.64). Fraiberg (1972), in her analyses of both girls and adult women, described images such as "an inferno" (p.440), "an explosion" (p.440), "a volcano" (p.460), and a "big wave" (p.463) from which there was no escape. The uncontrollable excitement produces great anxiety and a motive for inhibition of erotic sensation. The so-called "silent vagina" of girlhood is reflected in these patients' emotional deadness and lack of affect. Kramer (1954) reported the memories of a 36-year-old woman in the later stages of analysis. As a child of almost three years old, she recalled masturbating by inserting her finger into her vagina while looking into a mirror. At the sight of her own image she experienced strong vaginal contractions which were extremely frightening. This seemed a turning point in her childhood, after which she suppressed all temptation to masturbate.

A similar image of overwhelming excitement and terror was related to me by a woman in her 30s, who had been sexually assaulted in childhood, probably by her father. The patient recalled a story often told by her mother as a warning of the dangers of the outside world: a woman was taking a car trip with some of her friends though she was implored by her family not to go. The car was struck by a semi and burst into flames. Observers saw the women beating with their fists on the windows, trying to get out. Because of the shatterproof glass, they were unable to do so and were burned beyond recognition.

The story has haunted the woman throughout her life. In the treatment its significance became apparent. Her associations reflected both early sexual stimulation and the trapped and terrifying feelings of being assaulted. The "semi" was the adult male assailant. This is a particularly apt metaphor for this patient who has in the past experienced a driving phobia arising, I believe, out of the sexualization of driving experiences.

In addition to overwhelming fears and anxieties which may result in flight or denial of the vagina, Barnett (1966) pointed to factors relating to andiomical structure, location, and function which contribute to the repression of this organ. Barnett stated: "There is evidence that the vagina receives stimulation and that the vaginal introitus is manipulated in the neonate and infant girl. Memory traces of this activity are rarely, if ever, recoverable" (p.129). She suggested several hypotheses which could account for the repression of vaginal awareness on an intrapsychic level. First, because the orifice itself lacks voluntary muscle control, there is a continual threat to body integrity. Secondly, the vagina is difficult to incorporate into the body image because, unlike the mouth or anus, it has no contents which could be viewed as part of the self. Finally, as the result of the inability to maintain awareness of the vagina without anxiety, the organ is decathected and clitoral hypercathexis emerges to assist in vaginal repression.

The factors relating to the suppression of women's sexuality as reflected in vaginal awareness are innumerable. From an interpersonal and intrapsychic viewpoint, data suggest that the point of greatest impact on the developing female child is at the time of separation or individuation from the mother-child dyad. The mother-child dyad represents in microcosm the relationship of the female to the world around her. Like her mother's, her existence in-relation has seemingly more significance than her development as an individual. Yet she must also develop as an individual, gaining mastery over her own body just as the male child does. Beginning in the anal phase, this task often places her at odds with her loved mother, requiring an expression of aggression that is tolerated far less in female than in male children. Oliner (1982) stated furthermore that:

> the quality of the mother … makes it more difficult for the girl to attain mastery and individuality … The mother, being seen as more aggressive and intrusive, does not lend herself to being the suitable object of the girl's sadistic drive … and her ability to tolerate the girl's need for individuation is not experienced as reliable.
>
> (pp. 47–48)

It is the opinion of writers such as Oliner (1982), Kestenberg (1982), and David (1983) that the struggles of the anal phase have tremendous impact on the developmental tasks of the subsequent genital phase, particularly for the girl. Kestenberg and others have stated that anal and vaginal sensations are extremely difficult to differentiate and localize. Vaginal cathexis involves many of the same issues as anal mastery, such as loss of control, expression of aggression, and separation vis-a-vis the mother.

Relevant clinical data are provided by David (1983) who, by addressing these issues, successfully treated three adult women suffering from orgastic inhibition. All three women had hostile, disapproving mothers and were at the same time devalued as women by their fathers. Though oedipal issues were addressed, David stated that the symptoms of sexual dysfunction were relieved after issues related to "anal and urethral elimination, sadistic fantasies against both parents and their own sexual partners and fantasies of being robbed and injured while having sex" (p.10) were expressed, They began to process the aggression directed particularly toward their mothers and "to accept themselves, particularly their sexual selves" (p.11). They were finally able to achieve via the transference a separation from their mothers that they had never fully resolved.

In their discussion of a preoedipal genital phase, Glover and Mendell (1982) also focused on the often difficult task the little girl faces as she attempts to differentiate her own sexual identity while still relating to her mother, a same-sex person. In their small scale study, they identified four feminine styles in the mothers and the effects which they had on the daughters' efforts to separate from them. The authors also discussed the girl's view of the father as it impacts her development in the preoedipal genital phase. It is problematic, however, that although they viewed the mothers as realistically thwarting the girls' growing independence, the fathers' perceived sexual aggression was seen as existing only in fantasy. Though I am proposing that the little girl's sexual identity centered in early and continuing vaginal awareness is often at risk vis-a-vis her separation from her mother, I do not intend this as yet another instance of mother-blaming. Rather, I see it as part of a larger problem inherent in the mother-daughter relationship in a society which simultaneously depends on women as mothers and is threatened by women as individuals.

Why is the concept of vaginal awareness so controversial? Why is vaginal repression encountered so frequently that we have assumed it to be part of normal female development? Why are the data around vaginal excitation, awareness, and anxiety so difficult to recover? Why has there been such resistance to incorporating the data that we do have into a coherent theory of female development? Why are we so reluctant to assume that vaginal sensation, frequently enough reported by little girls, may represent a cathexis of the organ, an actual mental representation, as Glover and Mendell (1982) suggested, possibly experienced as "vaginal desire"? The answers to these questions as I have tried to show, lie in a complex mix of biological, cultural, and intrapsychic factors which have seemingly conspired to suppress women's individual expression of sexuality, viewed both as a threat to patriarchy and to her central role in the continuation of the species. It is woman as individual, an experiencing subject, with needs, desires, and impulses which she may or may not be able to control, who presents the greatest threat both to the world view and to the demanding infant in all of us. Like the penis, widely accepted as a symbol of male or phallic power, the female vagina, the primary organ of both reproductive and individual self-expression, has deep significance at individual and cultural levels as a symbol of female power. Its repression, both in individual women and men and at cultural levels, is an expression of our denial and fear of that power.

In conclusion, I have tried to show that the barriers to our understanding of the feminine unconscious are many and formidable but not insurmountable. Unless, however, we recognize that the roots of our resistance are not only cultural and intrapsychic but also biological and evolutionary, we will fail to comprehend the depth and intensity of our opposition, lying deep within our struggle to survive as a species. Vital to the preservation of the race, woman's awesome reproductive powers have been de-personified. She is nature, a cog in an evolutionary machine, subservient to maternity, without a will or decision-making capability of her own. At a psychological level she is the presence who bears us, suckles us, rocks us, and, as such, may have no needs or fantasies which differ from those of the demanding child within each of us. Finally, it is almost inconceivable that she should have a sexual life involving independent initiative and desire quite possibly unrelated to reproduction. Because humans are the first mammalian species in which the female does not go into heat, woman's inordinate and continuing sexual needs have had to be ruthlessly and universally subjugated to ensure her role in bearing and caring for children, as well as to establish paternity. As Sherfey stated, "although … couched in superstitious, religious and rationalized terms, behind the subjugation of women's sexuality lay the inexorable economics of cultural evolution which finally forced men to impose it and women to endure it" (1966, p.128). As we probe the depths of woman's physical and psychological interior, we strike deeply rooted and culturally sanctioned taboos ostensibly created to preserve our physical and psychological survival.

In recent times, however, we have begun to face the illusory nature of our beliefs about women, and about men as well. It is an illusion to assume that the human male exists at the center of our universe; that libido is male in origin; that woman is a benign presence lacking in independent thought or action; that we have achieved a victory of the intellect over the senses, or that we would want to do so; or, finally, that any of us exist without deep connections to those around us, connections of which we may or may not be aware. Illusions, as we know, do not serve us well. They are what Freud called:

> … a store of ideas … born from man's need to make his helplessness tolerable and built up from the material of memories of the helplessness of his own childhood and the childhood of the human race … the possession of these ideas protects him in two directions—against the dangers of nature and Fate, and against the injuries that threaten him from human society itself.
>
> (1927, p.18)

Like a childhood neurosis, our beliefs about the relative roles of women and men are born of wish fulfillment, resistant to data and experience which would prove otherwise. Only as we emerge however from the childhood of the race, bringing into conscious awareness the totality of human experience, will we achieve a triumph of human reason and a liberation of human spirit.

References

Barnett, M. (1966). Vaginal awareness in the infancy and childhood of girls. *Journal of the American Psychoanalytic Association*, *14*, 129–141.

Benedek, T. (1960). Organization of the reproductive drive. *International Journal of Psychoanalysis*, *41*, 1–15.

Brenner, C. (1976). *Psychoanalytic technique and psychic conflict*. New York: International Universities Press.

Chasseguet-Smirgel, J. (1976). Freud and female sexuality: The consideration of some blind spots in the exploration of the 'dark continent'. *International Journal of Psychoanalysis*, *37*, 275–286.

Chehrazi, S. (1986). Female psychology. *Journal of the American Psychoanalytic Association*, *34*, 141–162.

Chodorow, N. (1978). *The Reproduction of Mothering: Psychoanalysis and the Sociology of Gender*. Berkeley: University of California Press.

Chodorow, N. (1989). *Feminism and psychoanalytic theory*. New Haven, CT: Yale University Press.

David, C. (1983, July). An approach to understanding and treating orgastic inhibition. Paper presented at the *Michigan Society for Psychoanalytic Psychology, Summer Institute*, Traverse City, MI.

de Beauvoir, S. (2011). *The Second Sex*. New York: Vintage Books.

Deutsch, H. (1969). The psychology of woman in relation to the functions of reproduction. In Fliess (Ed.), *The Psychoanalytic Reader* (pp. 165–179). New York: International Universities Press.

Eissler, K. (1977). Comments on penis envy. *The Psychoanalytic Study of the Child*, *32*.

Fraiberg, S. (1972). Some characteristics of genital arousal and discharge in latency. *The Psychoanalytic Study of the Child*, *27*, 439–475.

Freud. S. (1905). Three essays on the theory of sexuality. 7, 125–245.

Freud, S. (1917). Introductory lectures on psychoanalysis. 15, 16.

Freud, S. (1927). The future of an illusion. 21, 3–56.

Freud, S. (1930). Civilization and its discontents. 21, 59–145.

Freud, S. (1931). Female sexuality. 21, 223–243.

Freud, S. (1933) New Introductory lectures on psychoanalysis. 22, 3–182.

Freud, S. (1939). Moses and monotheism. 23, 3–137.

Fromm-Reichmann, F. & Gunst, V.K. (1969). On the denial of women's sexual pleasure. In R. Fliess (Ed.). *The Psychoanalytic Reader* (pp. 75–84). New York: International Universities Press.

Gilligan, C. (1982). *In a Different Voice*. Cambridge, MA: Harvard University Press.

Glover. L. & Mendell, D. (1982). A suggested developmental sequence for a preoedipal genital phase. In D. Mendell (Ed.). *Early Female Development* (pp. 127–174). New York: Spectrum.

Goldstein, R. (1984). The dark continent and its enigmas. *International Journal of Psychoanalysis*, *65*, 179–189.

Greenacre, P. (1950). Problems of early female sexual development. *The Psychoanalytic Study of the Child*, *5*, 12–138.

Harris, A.E. (1985). Discussion. *Contemporary Psychoanalysis*, *21*, 17–25.

Horney, K. (1933). The denial of the vagina: Contribution to genital anxiety specific to women. *International Journal of Psychoanalysis*, *14*, 57–70.

Jones, E. (1927). The early development of female sexuality. *International Journal of Psychoanalysis*, *8*, 459–472.

Jordan, J. (1989). Relational development: Therapeutic implications of empathy and shame. *Work in Progress*, *39*.

Kaplan, E. A. (1983). *Women and Film: Both Sides of the Camera*. New York: Methuen.

Kestenberg, J. S. (1968). Outside and inside, male and female. *Journal of the American Psychoanalytic Association*, *16*, 457–519.
Kestenberg, J. (1975). *Children and Parents: Psychoanalytic Studies*. New York: Aronson.
Kestenberg, J. (1982). The inner-genital phase—Prephallic and preoedipal. In D. Mendell (Ed.), *Early Female Development* (pp. 81–126). New York: Spectrum.
Kleeman, J. (1976). Freud's early views. *Journal of the American Psychoanalytic Association*, *24*, 3–27.
Kramer, P. (1954). Early capacity for orgastic discharge and character formation. *The Psychoanalytic Study of the Child*, *9*, 128–141.
Kulish, N. (1990, January). The mental representation of the clitoris. Paper presented at a *Scientific meeting of the Michigan Psychoanalytic Society*, Southfield, MI.
Leavy, S. (1985). The rules of the game. *Contemporary Psychoanalysis*, *21*, 1–17.
Lerner, H. (1976). Parental mislabeling of female genitals as a determinant of penis envy and learning inhibitions in women. *Journal of the American Psychoanalytic Association*, *24*, 269–283.
Masters, W. H. & Johnson, V. (1966). *Human Sexual Response*. Boston: Little, Brown.
Miller, J.B. (1976). *Toward a New Psychology of Women*. Boston: Beacon.
Mitchell, J. (1975). *Psychoanalysis and Feminism*. New York: Vintage.
Mitchell, J. (1984). *Women: The Longest Revolution*. New York: Pantheon.
Montgrain, R. (1983). On the vicissitudes of female sexuality. The difficult path from anatomical destiny to psychic representation. *International Journal of Psychoanalysis*, *65*, 169–186.
Oliner, M. (1982). The anal phase. In D. Mendell (Ed.). *Early Female Development* (pp. 25–60). New York: Spectrum.
Rich, A. (1976). *Of Women Born*. New York: Norton.
Roheim, G. (1945). Aphrodite or the woman with a penis. *Psychoanalytic Quarterly*, *14*, 350–390.
Schafer, R. (1973). Problems in Freud's psychology of women. *Journal of the American Psychoanalytic Association*, *22*, 459–485.
Sherfey, M.J. (1966). The evolution and nature of female sexuality in relation to psychoanalytic theory. *Journal of the American Psychoanalytic Association*, *14*, 28–128.
Stoller, R. (1975). *Perversion: The Erotic Form of Hatred*. New York: Pantheon.
Tenbusch, L. G. (1987, March). Portrayal of women in film. Paper presented at a *meeting of the Association for Women in Psychology*, Washington, DC.
Thompson, C. (1969). Some effects of the derogatory attitude toward female sexuality. In R. Fliess (Ed.). *The Psychoanalytic Reader* (pp. 65–74). New York: International Universities Press.

Thompson, P. (1977). Locus of control, body articulation and sexual differentiation in women as modified by self-help and sex education programs. Unpublished doctoral dissertation. Michigan State University, Lansing, MI.

Westcott, M. (1986). *The Feminist Legacy of Karen Horney*. New Haven, CT: Yale University Press.

Wrye, H. (1983). The maternal erotic transference. Paper presented at the *spring meeting of the American Psychological Association. Division 39*. New York.

Chapter Two
The Therapist's Maternal Capacity

In this chapter I address the transference and countertransference that may exist with the nonverbal patient. Thus I endeavor to provide insight into the ways in which therapists and mothers alike may experience relationships with preverbal and nonverbal persons. The case study of Sarah illustrates my countertransference reactions in working with this traumatized and largely nonverbal young woman. In later stages of treatment Sarah began to express the wish that I would hold her hand and, for a few sessions, I did so. We ostensibly made a mutual decision to stop, but her demands continued, seemingly endlessly. Her interpersonal pressure for me to do so made the last five minutes of the sessions seem "interminable". She would even threaten suicide which had been a real possibility in the beginning of her treatment. In the context of this volume I can liken my feelings of desperation to the mothering experience in which it feels as though we can never meet the needs of our child for holding, attention, and engagement.

The article identifies three possible countertransference reactions, including "grandiose fantasies" that would imply that the patient/baby will be "reborn" as the result of our ministrations; the experience of the patient/baby wish for "boundariless fusion"; and the sensation of holding the patient/baby inside one's own body. It is important to recognize, however, that while the therapist's countertransference with the

DOI: 10.4324/9781003413677-3

nonverbal patient bears a resemblance to that of the mother with her preverbal child, there are important differences. The mother may be on call 24/7; she is unpaid; and she is, quite literally, responsible for the survival of her child in a way that a therapist is not.

The article begins with the recognition of theoretical development and clinical experience over the past 20 years that have come increasingly to recognize a group of pathologies whose onset occurs in the early developmental period of the child, before language and before significant structural differentiation has taken place. These pathologies, involving developmental arrests and deficits in the core structure of the self, have necessitated a revision or certainly an extension of classical theory and technique. We have come to recognize that crucial reparative work must frequently be done and that this work must take place within the context of a relationship which provides the kind of empathic attunement that was missing in the original mother/infant experience. The psychoanalytic therapist, like the good mother, must furnish a safe space, a holding environment, in which the patient's maturational needs can unfold. For those patients who evidence these early developmental deficits, the traditional tools of psychoanalysis, that is, free association and verbal or representational exploration of the transference relationship, are not readily available. These patients must first experience the "being," the holding, the confirmation of their continuous existence, much of which must be communicated nonverbally, before the symbolic conflict-based work can proceed.

Our work in this area, once thought to be outside the domain of psychoanalysis, has been greatly facilitated by the convergence of several lines of discourse which I wish to touch upon briefly. Our understanding of the early mother/child relationship, for example, has been greatly expanded by the explosion of research which has revolutionized our view of the infant.

Observational research from many quarters has taught us that from the moment of birth the intelligent infant is an engaging, hard-working being, striving within the limits of its physical capabilities to interact with the caregiver and thereby influence its human environment. The notion of a passive, encapsulated, nearly autistic phase has given way to the realization that from birth on the infant has the capacity to synthesize experience and arrange an ever-widening and complex assortment of stimuli. What has emerged from our greatly increased understanding of this early phase of life is a realization of the extraordinary complexity of the mother/infant relationship. Though the communication is largely non-verbal, certainly on the part of the infant, mother and child are found to be engaging in a complex continuing social dialogue, one which is absolutely crucial in the formation of a human being. Insofar as we attempt to replicate aspects of this early relationship in the clinical setting, we must acknowledge that a significant part of the communication between therapist and patient will be, at least initially, in nonverbal form.

A second and related line of thought has been what Stolorow calls "the shift from drive to affect as the central motivational construct for psychoanalysis" (1992, p.26). As Stolorow points out, affective development is not a product of isolated intrapsychic mechanisms but a property of the child/care-giver system of mutual regulation. Viewed from this perspective, the effectiveness of the therapist/analyst becomes heavily dependent upon the ability to resonate with the patient's affective states and respond, often cross-modally, with affective states of the therapist's own. In this type of emotional environment, again reminiscent of the original mother-infant bond, the patient may experience the kind of "vitality affects" (Stern, 1985) which generate a felt connection and ultimately, a cohesive sense of self.

A third and obviously related and highly influential line of thought, one which has the potential to increase our understanding of the "mothering" function, is the relatively recent acknowledgment that the mother herself is a subjective being with a perspective of her own. We have come to realize that the context in which the child matures, i.e. the "facilitating environment", is indeed occupied by a person, a woman with needs and desires which may or may not match those of the infant. As we shift our outlook to emphasize the *relationship* between mother and child, we recognize an interactive synchrony between two engaged individuals in alternating roles of subject and object, observer and observed. It is an interconnection which, at its best, becomes the prototype of mutuality, spontaneity, and authenticity in all relationships to come. The analytic engagement then, insofar as it partakes of that primal bond, becomes a living, interactive drama in which two participants, therapist and patient, strive to co-create those experiences of reciprocity, mutual recognition, and intimacy which facilitate change.

The convergence of these three lines of discourse—our new understanding of the intelligent infant; the importance of affect in the development of the self; and the perspective on mothering as a subjective experience—has both widened the scope of pathology amenable to analytic treatment and altered our view of the analytic process itself. Work with those patients whose pathology involves developmental arrests and deficits in the core structure of the self becomes heavily dependent on the capacity of the psychoanalytic therapist to remain affectively attuned in ways that the original caregiver could not. The therapist is, in short, functioning in many respects as would a mother in providing a nurturing, sustaining relational medium in which her child may grow.

There are, of course, important differences. The similarities between the relationship of infant and caregiver and that of patient and therapist are many, the comparisons are frequent and apt. The mother/child relationship becomes the prototype for that between therapist and patient. As we attempt to broaden our understanding of this critical aspect of our clinical capabilities, it becomes appropriate to comprehend and describe as fully as possible the actual experience of mothering from the mother's own subjective point of view.

It is this line of inquiry which I wish to undertake through examination of the following questions: What precisely are mothers experiencing when they are responding empathically to their infants? How are they doing it? The question of why they are doing it is also important but well beyond the scope of this paper. Given that it is near-universal that women have mothered, how and to what extent are men able to access this kind of nonverbal receptivity and what are the special complications they face in doing so? How is this maternal capacity applied clinically in working with prerepresentational body-based transference? How does countertransference manifest itself in working with nonverbal material? Finally, I wish to present ongoing case material in which all of these issues have been particularly relevant.

WHO IS MOTHER?

How do we comprehend the experience of mothering from the mother's own subjective viewpoint? I believe that we must begin by acknowledging that it is frightening to attempt to do so. It is frightening because all of us, at some level, carry within us the memory and the mental image of ourselves as tiny infants, helpless in relation to mother's awesome power. Hirsch has accurately described this limitation within classical discourse.

> Mother ... remains absent even to herself. The place she inhabits is vacant. Although she produces and upholds the subject, she herself remains the matrix, the other, the origin ... Is it possible to tell the untold tale of maternal participation in the psychoanalytic narrative, staying

> within psychoanalytic terminology? Can we invest with speech the silence that defines maternal experience?
> (1989, pp. 168–169)

Yet the psychoanalytic imperative to bring the unconscious into consciousness impels us forward. We have traveled into forbidden zones before and can do it again as we explore, this time from both sides, the earliest bond.

With notable exceptions such as the work of Daniel Stern, descriptions of the mother/infant relationship from the mother's perspective have focused solely on her symbolic and representational world, particularly as it affects her infant. Early work such as that of Winnicott (1957, 1965) and Wilfred Bion (1967) outline the fantasy life of the mother and her reveries, preoccupations, and projective identifications involving the infant. Fraiberg, Adelson, and Shapiro placed maternal fantasies of a pathogenic nature at the core of disturbed parent/infant relationships with her concept of "ghost in the nursery" (1975). In recent years an explosion of psychoanalytic research has also focused on the maternal representational world but, though these studies are highly illuminating, they do not tell us how these representations are translated into actual behavior.

Yet it is precisely the "doing" which interests us, The infant does not know or care what the mother is thinking except insofar as it affects what she is doing with him or to him. For those of us who are trying to understand what is unique about mothering, it is the "doing", manifest in moment-by-moment interactions of mother and child, that distinguishes it surely as much as the thinking. It is the mother's inner world, as it is translated into hundreds of behavioral acts, that ultimately communicates with the child. Again, Stern acknowledges the impact of maternal fantasy upon the infant but says that there is no "ether medium" through which fantasies of mother and infant could affect each other unless they take a form that is perceivable and discriminable to both.

One of the significant difficulties in describing this experience from the mother's point of view is that it is for her, as well as for the baby; a phenomenon which is largely nonverbal and physically encoded. As described by Wrye and Welles, it is mother and baby in close physical contact.

> The infant, having once been literally encapsulated in mother's womb in amniotic fluid, experiences closeness postnatally through contact with skin and bodily fluids,

> through her caretaking in relation to milk, drool, urine, feces, mucus, spit, tears, and perspiration. A mother's contact with and ministrations to her baby in dealings with these fluids may optimally create a slippery, sticky sensual adhesion in the relationship; it is, so to speak, the medium for bonding. This sensuality, experienced by both parties, is key in their relationship.
>
> (1994, p.35)

It is from within this slippery, sticky, sensual, and nonverbal bond that mother and baby create their dance of reciprocity and engagement.

Yet as Stern (1985, 1995) has pointed out, the mother's experiences, as well as those of the nonverbal infant, appear to remain largely outside of consciousness. She seems unable even to begin to describe what she is doing, what it feels like, and how she accomplishes it, It has remained in that realm of human experience occupied by the poetic, the spiritual, and the mystical. Stern's pioneering work has represented a monumental effort to bring that realm of human experience into consciousness through his painstaking descriptions in behavioral terms of the hundreds of actions and interactions which comprise the mother/child relationship. He describes this early bond as characterized by an infinite number of lived, moment-by-moment, largely nonverbal, experiences which, taken together over days, weeks, months, and years, form the individual representations of their life together. The mother's effective participation in this critical period in the child's life rests on her ability to read and respond appropriately to the cues which the child gives. Stern (1995) suggests that these daily acts of mothering evoke memories of the mother's infancy and of the mothering she received from her own mother. It requires a kind of "empathic immersion and primary identification" (1995, p.181) which may never have been fully employed before.

The mother's stored memories include both sides of the interaction, that is, the parts that she experienced directly as a baby, and the parts of her mother's experience that she felt empathically through imitation and primary identification. Except in pathological situations, this need not necessitate regression. It involves access, possibly unconscious or preconscious, to the mother's own functioning in infancy and, through identification, to that of her mother. It entails access to a play space or transitional space into which she can enter, reside comfortably without getting lost, and eventually leave in order to return to her already highly organized representational world.

Through Stern's intricate descriptions, however, we are able to understand the mothering experience, previously thought of as intuitive or even instinctual, in terms of micro-events. These are distinct from macro-events which occupy most clinical theories, such as the birth of a sibling, the mother's emotional availability, and so on. The clinical analysis of micro-events involves questions such as the following: What is the physical distance between the partners? What is the physical orientation—turned toward the side or full-facing? Where are the eyes looking? Is there mutual gaze? How loud or soft are the vocalizations? It clearly illustrates that it is not just the baby's reaction to the mother, but also the mother's reaction to the baby, which creates their relationship.

Stern suggest that the mother's capability to respond to the needs of her infant arises out of a unique psychic organization which he calls the "motherhood constellation" (1995). He identifies several themes which emerge when a woman becomes a mother in our culture. The first, called the life-growth theme, involves the following basic question: Can the mother keep the baby alive? Can she make the baby grow and thrive physically? He adds that this theme is unique in the life cycle and I would add that it is unique to women. There are no other comparable relationships or points in the life cycle where one person is responsible for the life and growth of another.

The second, called the primary-relatedness theme, involves the mother's social-emotional engagement with the baby. Can mother love the baby? Can she feel that the baby loves her? Can she realize that this is truly her baby? Stern states that this concept of primary relatedness concerns the very essence of what it means to be human, including the establishment of basic human ties of attachment, security, and affection.

Again, I would add that this type of relationship is also unique in the life cycle. The work of early mothering literally transforms a biological organism into a human being. I believe that it is the influence of these two themes which creates the singular quality of the mother/infant relationship. Furthermore, their primal urgency ensures the kind of avoidance and denial which has made it so difficult to explain in terms of simple human behavior.

Winnicott's concept of "primary maternal preoccupation" (1957) is similar to that of the motherhood constellation, particularly the primary relatedness theme. He states that soon after conception is known to have taken place the woman begins to "shift some of her sense of self on to the baby that is growing within her" (1965, p.53). Through projective identification with the baby, the mother is able to achieve a powerful sense of what the baby needs.

Interestingly enough, Winnicott also draws a comparison between the mother and the analyst who is attempting to meet the needs of a patient who is reliving these very early stages in the transference. He states that the analyst goes through changes in orientation which are similar to those of the mother but that "the analyst, *unlike the mother*, needs to be aware of the sensitivity which develops in him or her in response to the patient's immaturity and dependence" (1965, p.53; my italic). While he acknowledges that it is important and useful to understand maternal sensitivity, he continues to overlook the subjective state of the mother.

It is my belief that while certain aspects of mothering may alter in intensity during crucial phases, the fact that women can mother and universally have mothered, is a critical organizing factor in their psychic lives. It is a fact which prevails whether they have actually given birth or not. I further believe that women's reproductive capabilities are a central organizing aspect of their psycho-sexual development. I do not wish to enter at this point the current debate about the constructionist versus essentialist, fluid versus fixed nature of gender. While I feel that it is a useful debate and relevant to this topic, my purpose for this paper is to explore those aspects of mothering which are pertinent in the clinical setting. In doing so, I cannot ignore the obvious fact that it is women who have mothered throughout human history. Furthermore, "new" fathers notwithstanding, the experience for most of us and for most of our patients was that of being cared for as infants by women. As Ruddick states, to assume that mothering is genderless, "trivializes both the distinctive costs of mothering to women as well as the effects, for worse and for better, of femininity on maternal practice and thought" (1989, p.xiii). The survival of their children and of the species itself has depended on their becoming skilled at what they do. I believe that it is unreasonable to assume that this activity which has occupied the vast majority of women for the bulk of their adult lives for thousands of years has not greatly influenced their unique development.

Does this indicate that only women can mother? Does it mean that mothering is innate, biologically given, informed solely by the anatomical and hormonal differences between men and women? Probably not, but then again these are the very questions I am attempting to explore. Insofar as we can examine this aspect of human behavior and bring it into the critical light of day, we can apply our knowledge, not only in the clinical setting, but also in the deconstruction of rigid and limiting gender stereotypes.

In summary, when we speak about mothering we are talking about a specific set of behaviors, performed historically only by women and based upon their own experience of being mothered as infants. It is unique in the human life cycle and, when viewed in terms of the kind of skill and commitment required, it is truly an amazing feat. It is this unique constellation of attributes and sensitivities which we as therapists profess to bring into the clinical setting for those patients who are reliving very early stages in the transference. How do we accomplish this? Can we describe in a conscious and relatively systematic way our experiences in doing so? Do we, for example, feel the kind of life-and-death urgency in regard to our patients which a mother, of necessity, feels for her child, and what are the costs to us if we do? How and to what extent are men able to provide the kind of attunement which mothering entails and what are the particular difficulties they face in doing so?

HOW DO MEN MOTHER?

In this discussion we have been viewing aspects of the infant/mother bond as an analogue for the therapist/patient relationship. The therapist's capacity to provide the kind of psychobiological attunement that was missing in the relationship with the early caregiver is critical for those patients with ruptures in the affective core of the self. Yet, in reality, across human history it is women who have provided this, Father's relationship to the infants has typically been quite different. Furthermore, we who are therapists as well as our adult patients were, almost without exception, raised by women.

If we take the position that, given thousands of years of evolution, female primates (including women) may have a biologically-based substratum of mothering responses, but that the complex interaction between mother and infant is still heavily influenced by social learning and individual experience, we may then assume that men can indeed access their maternal capacity. Their ability to do so would, to a large extent, depend on their comfort with their own maternal and feminine identification. It is this point of view that I would like to discuss in this paper.

Parenthetically I would add a third perspective, one which I find both illogical and disturbing, which holds that while both men and women can access mothering skills and capabilities whenever necessary, it is only women who should continue to do the actual mothering.

From a developmental perspective, the male child begins to consolidate his gender identity at roughly the same time he is acquiring verbal and symbolic skills. He recognizes that the concept male, even as he dimly comprehends it, specifically states "not mother" as one of its defining characteristics. While the little boy may continue to share his internal feeling states with his mother, both verbally and nonverbally, he, unlike the little girl, must, albeit unconsciously, decline to identify with that aspect of his mother which understands them.

Mother provides an emotional holding environment through which the child's own inner states may be reflected, understood, and shared. It is an atmosphere of safety which she provides for exploring, experiencing, and feeling in the world and which the child comes, through identification, to be able to provide for himself. When that identification is disallowed, the child or adult must search for and depend on others to provide the emotional holding. Plus the male, lacking in varying degrees this feminine identification, may be unable to access his own inner feeling states or attune to and share inner affective states with another.

In the clinical setting the male therapist or analyst may be called upon to provide the kind of emotional holding or attunement needed by patients who are reliving these early preverbal experiences in the transference. The male therapist may fail to recognize or acknowledge this type of material in defense against what Wrye and Welles call "regressive immersion in boundariless erotic fusion" (1994, p.85) if he is without access to or heavily defended against his own maternal identification. Without recoiling in anxiety, the analyst must be able to permit himself to experience a range of primitive and sensual body states engendered by the patient's material. He must be able to tolerate the fear that overwhelming anxiety will flood him, pull him away from analytic composure, erode professional boundaries, and threaten his masculine identity. When the pathology is severe and self-other differentiation is not well-established, the threat of annihilation anxiety and regression into the mother's body evokes sheer terror on both sides of the couch.

THE PRE-REPRESENTATIONAL TRANSFERENCE

Transference as we traditionally think of it rests on the individual's ability to formulate mental representation. A person can put into words various thoughts, feelings, and wishes, elaborate themes and patterns, and explore their connections and relationships. Oedipal transferences involve triangular conflicts around sexuality and aggression. Pre-oedipal transferences concern issues of anger, dependency, separation, and control. The patient's ability to work with these issues, including the abstraction of emotion, in symbolic form, is the means for exploring it.

In pre-representational transference, however, the elements are far less obvious and are grounded in preverbal levels of development. Quite distinct from verbal productions, the patient may be concerned with very basic issues having to do with self-regulation, safety, security, and attachment. As Krystal (1988) and McDougall (1989) point out, affects may be in their early form in which they are experienced as body sensations, resulting in alexithymic and psychosomatic conditions and disorders.

The successful treatment of the pre-representational transference rests with the therapist's ability to provide a holding environment, a safe space in which the patient's maturational needs can unfold. The therapist must function, in many ways, as a real object, one who can provide the kind of emotional validation that affirms the patient's continuous existence in ways that were not available in the early environment. In order for this reparative work to move forward, the patient cannot make do with the fantasy of empathy, but must experience real empathy. The patient must perceive the therapist's real emotional availability, affective attunement, and nonsterile holding. In the context of a relationship which acknowledges and addresses the deficits experienced early in life, the patient will then begin to repair structural ruptures and will become increasingly able to ally with the therapist in an investigative attitude which will allow the exploration of the meaning of thoughts, feelings, wishes, and behavior.

Of course, in practice the theoretical differences which distinguish a pre-representational transference from a. traditional one are often difficult to discern. The task of the therapist is, as Killingmo states, to "derive his therapeutic strategy from an understanding of the unique structural make-up of the patient and formulate and apply his interventions so that they match this very structure" (1989, p.66).

This is, after all, exactly what a good mother would do, i.e., match her responses and interventions to acknowledge the developing capabilities of her child.

I wish now to focus on three developmental levels of communication and relatedness which may present themselves in the pre-representational transference and which must be brought to some resolution before the more traditional transference work may occur.

The earliest developmental level is identified by Greenspan (1989) as the level of engagement. It is drawn from the birth to two-month period where the essential tasks of the infant-mother relationship are the organization and regulation of elemental sleep-wake cycles, feeding patterns, and management of stimulus input as well as soothing and self-soothing behavior usually involving contact with the mother's body, breathing patterns, and heart-rate. The level of engagement also includes the period from two to approximately seven months where interaction becomes noticeably more social. It is here that the individual is making vital connections to the human world as the source of comfort, interest, pleasure, and joy, as well as the provider of physical needs.

There are wide discrepancies in the extent to which engagement is an issue in the treatment setting depending, of course, on the level of pathology involved. I believe that it is a significant factor in many treatments, particularly in the beginning stages, and that it is frequently overlooked because it is communicated at the nonverbal level. Of course neither the sociopathic nor extremely withdrawn individual make it into the consulting room, at least voluntarily. We have, however, encountered the very frightened or anxious patient, barely able to sit in a chair or make eye contact. We sit in our chairs, ourselves barely able to move lest we scare them off, and struggle to interact in a way that is neither too intrusive nor too aloof.

I am reminded of such a patient, a 26-year-old woman, who had already been in treatment for over three years when I was forced precipitously to move my office when the clinic where I was working suddenly closed. I had indicated that she should follow me down the hall to my office. I walked down the hallway, assuming that she would follow, but she did not appear. I went back and found her frozen in the spot where I had left her. We then walked slowly together back to my office and it was only after she had visually examined the hallway, the office, and virtually every object in it that she was able to speak at all.

The second developmental level, that of gestural communication, comes from the childhood period of about nine to eighteen months. Infant researchers and observant parents are keenly aware of a dramatic shift which takes place in the infant at around nine months. Stern (1985) states that it is at this point that babies seem to sense that they have an inner subjective life of their own and that others do as well. It is now not enough for mommy to do things for them. She must also be able to share the focus of their attention, interest, and pleasure. The infant is, of course, still unable to communicate verbally, so, as Greenspan points out (1989), the mother and baby develop an elaborate system of nonverbal signaling. The infant is moving from the primarily proximal mode of relating based on physical holding and bodily contact to the distal modes involving nods, gestures, and eye contact, even across the room. Stern and Greenspan both emphasize that this ability to signal and communicate about inner feelings and intentions is a vital precursor to representational communication.

Greenspan further points out that some of the most basic emotional messages of life are communicated at the gestural level. Critical information such as safety versus danger, acceptance versus rejection, concern versus indifference, acceptance versus control, and respect versus humiliation are communicated presymbolically. When this particular mode has not been mastered, a person who seems to be communicating verbally may in fact be assessing issues of rejection, danger, or safety at a nonverbal level.

Stern states that much of the attunement which goes on at this develop mental level is not about categorical affects such as anger, surprise, joy, etc. Rather, it is an apprehension of what he calls "'vitality affects", qualities which he describes as "surging, fading away, fleeting, explosive, crescendo, decrescendo, bursting … and so on" (1985, p.54). A patient of mine, who has struggled for a long time to articulate her feeling states, recently described what she said was a "whoosh" feeling. I believe it is often these vitality affects that we are trying to comprehend when we feel particularly befuddled by our feeling experience with a patient.

Our lack of attention to the importance of the gestural level of communication is often, I believe, a contributing factor in failures in empathy, in abrupt terminations, or in therapies that never get going at all. I recall a man in his late twenties who had entered treatment largely at the urging of his wife who was about to leave him. He lacked verbal skills but seemed to be making a genuine effort to enter into treatment. After only a few sessions, he came into the office on a very warm day, wearing a black leather jacket elaborately decorated with silver zippers and grommets. It appeared to be brand new and very expensive. Toward the middle of the session in which he must have been sweltering he said, "I guess I'll take this thing off". He then slowly and deliberately removed the jacket. The session ended and he did not return to therapy. With hindsight I realized that, while there were surely other contributing factors, a significant reason that he did not return was because I had missed the nonverbal statement that he was making with the jacket. He was telling me something about himself, his unique characteristics, perhaps his masculinity, the way in which he loved himself, which I failed to acknowledge. Had I picked up on this nonverbal communication and responded empathically, the outcome might have been different.

Finally, I believe that the gestural level of communication must be attended to even with those patients who are communicating at predominantly verbal levels. We must keep in constant awareness questions such as the following: Where does the patient wait in the waiting room? How does the patient walk? What is communicated with posture or manner of dress? Is eye contact made before lying down on the couch? Is eye contact made in face-to-face therapy? When the timing is appropriate to bring into conscious and verbal awareness this very significant nonverbal communication, the patient is far better able to understand the meaning of his or her behavior and make informed decisions about how to change its problematic aspects.

The third and final level of development which I want to consider draws from the period beginning around 18 months when the child is becoming verbal. In ideal circumstances the child would begin to communicate in symbolic ways about shared meanings and feeling states and would be increasingly able to distinguish fantasy from reality, differentiate inner subjective experience from external occurrences, and connect events and feeling states and put them into sequence or context. But because of problems in earlier phases of engagement and gestural communication, this capacity may be greatly compromised so that the person is actually functioning at a level that we might term behavioral description. The patient describes physical events or behavioral events but cannot abstract emotional states. The therapist might mistakenly believe that the person understands the appropriate feeling state and might in fact supply it. If, for example, the patient says "I hit my boss," the therapist might respond, "You must have felt angry". If this interpretation is premature and the individual is not functioning at a truly representational level, he will be mystified by the comment. If being compliant, the patient may even agree but this will not move the process forward. If the whole procedure appears stagnated; if descriptions of external events are repeated over and over in unchanged form; and particularly, if typical kinds of transference interpretations fall on deaf ears, it is likely that the individual is using language in a purely descriptive way, without the capacity for interpersonal emotional exchange.

This was clarified for me in my work with a very intellectualized man in his early thirties who has been in once-a-week treatment for about seven years. He is extremely logical, verbal, and intelligent, and has an advanced degree in a highly scientific field. When he first began treatment he was able to describe detailed sequences of events which had transpired between him and his wife in particular. He was, however, unable to talk about or apparently understand the feeling states, either in himself or others, which might accompany those events. Over time, as we have gone over behavioral sequences in minute detail, stopping the action at many points to ascertain what he or another person might have been experiencing, this has changed. He has, in the context of an environment where he feels increasingly safe to reveal himself, been able to abstract emotion. Recently he described how in the past he had been paralyzed into inaction because he knew in advance how his wife would react to what he might say or do. He said that he had previously thought of emotions as if they were the solution to a math problem. Once one had arrived at the solution it could never be changed. He now realizes that emotions are fluid and changing—like human beings. He has evolved to a new level of representational thinking where the possibilities for interpersonal exchange are indeed infinite.

Early developmental issues, as they evolve from tasks of self-regulation and engagement through gestural communication and behavioral description to true symbolic expression, are, of course, transacted through close, continuing, and intimate contact with the mother figure. The patient reworks the issues within the maternal transference. Wrye and Welles (1994) have coined the term "maternal erotic transference" to capture the highly sensual nature of this relationship, arising as it does from a time before words when the medium of communication was actual physical contact with the mother's body as well as ministrations by her to the body of the infant. Not only is communication nonverbal, but it is also messy, comprised as it is of various bodily fluids—milk, saliva, urine, mucous, feces—around which the mother-infant relationship is, of necessity, organized. Moreover it involves the kind of rocking, nursing, patting, holding, and stroking through which the infant's needs are met. It is these largely repressed experiences, both painful and pleasurable, which a patient, in the throes of a maternal erotic transference, attempts to recreate in an effort to re-work pre-representational developmental issues. I believe it is noteworthy that, although numerous analysts have written with great accuracy about the mother-infant bond, it is two women analysts who have, at least to my knowledge, first addressed this particular messy, sensual aspect of it as it appears in the clinical setting. The development of a maternal erotic transference is impelled by patient's desire for a transformational experience in and through body of the analyst. He or she feels invisible, perhaps dead inside, or a "horrible dry hollow" (Wrye and Welles, 1994). For these patients, the transformational aspect of the maternal erotic transference represents a creative attempt to "make the mother/therapist into a living, more dimensional whole person and thereby become alive himself" (p.40).

As the maternal erotic transference begins to develop, the patient's material may take on a monotonous, concrete quality. Killingmo (1989) describes qualities of both monotonous persistence (p.72) and directness in the patient's way of demanding. The free flow of associations, even from verbally articulate patients, becomes blocked or filled with pregnant pauses, or stuck. Words seem to be expelled rather than spoken. Bodily concerns become central and, if the patient is verbal enough, associations are filled with vivid body imagery. Wrye and Welles (1994), for example, describe a patient who would report the sensation of feces running down her leg or her analyst's leg. For patients who are not able to work symbolically, concern with these issues may take a variety of concrete forms of enactment, for example, being preoccupied with the therapist's office, furnishings, car, or clothing; bringing items into the consulting room to be "stored" or "safe"; bringing gifts; showing rather than telling. The patient may attack the analytic frame by missing sessions or refusing to pay. Though there may be many meanings to these enactments, Wrye and Welles stress the concrete quality as a common denominator. The patient, and perhaps the therapist, are experiencing something at a preverbal level that cannot be verbalized. The task of the therapist is to recognize the enactments for what they are, and remain in touch with his or her own responses without either distancing or acting out. The therapist may then endeavor to bring into conscious awareness the underlying issues in whatever form the patient is able to tolerate.

THE PRE-REPRESENTATIONAL COUNTERTRANSFERENCE

As we consider the pre-representational countertransference, we now focus on the subjective experience of the therapist working with preverbal body-based material in these patients who, due to developmental arrests, have limited capacity to express themselves in verbal abstract form. In order to expand our understanding of the experience of the therapist we must return to our original inquiry: What are mothers experiencing when they are responding empathically to their infants?

Again, of course, the usual caveats apply. We are not really responsible for raising our patients. Their lives don't literally depend on us (even if it sometimes feels like they do). Yet we acknowledge that there are important similarities. In order for this reparative work to occur we must respond empathically. We must reach out with our feelings and become involved. Yet as with the attuned mother, we must continuously ask ourselves: How do I do this while still respecting the child/patient's autonomy? For us as psychoanalytic therapists the questions become very specific: How do I become empathically involved without eroding professional boundaries? How do I do this and still maintain the psychoanalytic frame? These are very difficult questions. We tread a fine line and there are no easy answers.

Again I believe the solution lies in trying to comprehend what it is we are doing. We need to make as explicit, conscious, and systematic as possible the nonverbal body-based sensations, responses, and interventions which are necessitated by this type of material. We do this by closely monitoring both ourselves and our work, consulting with colleagues when needed, and listening to our patients and their responses to our interventions. When we take risks, we will inevitably make mistakes. But then again, if we don't take risks we won't be successful with this kind of work at all. As in the mother-child relationship, it is the empathic failures on the part of the therapist which provide the opportunity and motivation for needed internalization on the part of the patient. Mistakes and even enactments are unavoidable. As Wrye and Welles state, "it is not possible to experience a countertransference fully without minimally enacting it in the treatment" (1994, p.64).

In their discussion of countertransference Wrye and Welles (1994) also point out that the therapist's responses may or may not match or mimic those of patient. It is likely however that, at least initially, countertransference reactions will occur in nonverbal form. Unusual bodily responses—sleepiness, boredom, disinterest, apathy—all may signal that nonverbal material, out of conscious awareness of both patient and therapist, is emerging. The therapist may even be responding verbally, and yet, an outside observer or video tape recording would reveal rapid speech, angry tones, confusing body language, i.e., a parallel response to the chaotic nonverbal material presented by the patient. It is the kind of parallel nonverbal communication one might observe in parents' unwitting mimicry of the gestural language of their eighteen-to-twenty-month-old babies.

In their own work Wrye and Welles (1994) have identified three types of countertransference reactions. The first involves grandiose fantasies which emerge as feelings on the part of the therapist that the patient will be totally remade or reborn as a result of therapy. This may include the belief that some type of physical contact with the patient will be a magic cure. A second reaction which they have identified involves a depressive response to patient's need either for fusion or separation. Where the patient seeks fusion through regression, the therapist attempts to ward it off with crisp insights and penetrating interpretations, defensively refusing to be consumed. Conversely, when the patient is ready to separate, the therapist holds onto a view of the patient as infantilized, depressed, and needy. A third type of response occurs when the therapist distances themself from the patient's all-consuming demands which threaten to swallow up the therapist's office, home, and body. The therapist's disavowal of this type of material may in fact render the treatment lifeless.

In addition to these countertransference responses which block transformational work, Wrye and Welles also identify some aspects of therapist gender which may make it more difficult for therapists of one sex or the other to work with certain types of erotic transference material. They posit that female therapists may be able to identify and enter more easily into patients' wishes for boundariless fusion since it is less likely to threaten their female identity. Males, on the other hand, while finding it more difficult to tolerate the regression necessary for working with the maternal erotic transference, may more readily recognize the patients' oedipal sexual strivings toward them.

I would like to propose an additional factor, which is implied by a number of authors but nevertheless not explicitly spelled out, as a significant, even necessary, element of a therapist's response to a patient with early developmental deficits. I am referring to that aspect of mothering which Winnicott called "primary maternal preoccupation" (1957) and which Stern referred to as the "motherhood constellation" (1995). Though there are many elements to these concepts, the key feature which I want to address has to do with the mother's investment in the child. To grow and thrive, the child must become the apple of mother's eye. The mother must think about the child, indeed become preoccupied with it, unreasonably so. This investment, almost by definition, has a narcissistic quality to it. This must, of course, be monitored for the child's best interests, but it means that the child's delight is the mother's delight. Lacking this aspect the caregiving is perfunctory, even custodial. In the clinical setting without this element of concern, investment, unreasoning delight in the patient's growth and transformation, the treatment also becomes custodial, perhaps technically correct, but ultimately lifeless.

Finally, I would like to suggest some ways in which this particular feature of countertransference has become identifiable to me. First of all, in working with patients who are particularly regressed, I have become aware of the sensation of holding them inside me as if they were literally a baby in the womb. This concept, which was clarified for me by Koeple

(1996), recognizes the mother's original investment in the child as part of her own body. I believe that this facilitates, in ways which are not as yet clear to me, the kind of emotional holding which I can provide. As Koeple pointed out this kind of holding is possible, at least for women analysts, without overwhelming fears of regression or fragmentation. This may indeed be a key point in which men and women differ.

A second element which I believe to be critical in the therapist's investment in the patient has to do with a function which Stern named "interpersonal communion" (1985, p.148). This factor was identified by those mothers whom he studied as their primary reason or motivation for wanting to be attuned to their infants. It was their desire to be with the infant, to share the infant's experience with no attempt, at that moment, to change, restructure, or modify in any way what the child was doing or believing. By the same token, the attuned therapist must convey to the patient that there are times when they are doing nothing more nor less than being together in the moment.

A third aspect of this quality of investment in the child/patient is something I have identified as I have been working on this presentation. This is not the first time that a patient has made rather remarkable gains during the time that I have been preparing a paper or presentation about him or her. I have observed this phenomenon in the patient I will be presenting below and in others as well. There may, of course, be many factors involved here. I may be conveying at some unconscious level that I need the patient to improve in certain ways so that I can appear in a favorable light to colleagues. The additional work that I do in preparing the case, e.g., extraordinary efforts at formulation and clarification, may bring to light important features which enhance the treatment. But I believe that there is another factor which relates to the quality of investment which she experiences from me. During the time that I have been preparing this paper I have indeed| thinking about her an unusual amount. At times I have been nearly obsessed with her, with the case, and how I will present it. Isn't this the kind of unreasoning preoccupation and involvement that children long to have from their mothers? Children want and, in fact, need their mothers to hold in a mental image of them during periods when they are separated. It actually helps them, as I believe it does my patient, to maintain a continuous sense themselves. Other patients express this sentiment, though perhaps more circumspectly than my patient. I'm sure many of us have been asked, "Are you going to write a book about me?" I believe that this is a wish that many hold, i.e., to be kept in the mind of a beloved other as we once existed in the mind of our mother, and I believe that it has a reparative effect in the treatment situation.

SARAH, A CASE STUDY

Sarah, a single woman in her mid-thirties, initiated treatment because of problems she was having at work. She had great difficulty communicating with her supervisors and was in danger of being fired. She was also ending a relationship with a man who had begun seeing another woman before their relationship had ended. She was relatively isolated except for her contact with men and women who frequently used and occasionally sold drugs. She was a regular marijuana user and was also addicted to cigarettes and food. She also had and continues to have physical problems related to health habits.

The initial phases of treatment consisted of my attempt to provide a stable contact point for her as she struggled to manage her life. I was able to do little more than provide a secure and dependable holding environment consisting of regular twice weekly sessions, payments on time, attention to vacations, missed appointments, cancellations, etc. She seemed able to tolerate this and was aware of her need to keep coming though she couldn't articulate why.

During this period Sarah would frequently begin the sessions by attempting to read my moods and facial expressions, and would comment endlessly on my feeling states. It was as if her task in life was to assess others and adapt to them as best she could. Her other focus consisted of descriptions of the people and situations in her life which were often exploitive Any effort on my part to explore her own inner reactions to these situations or her responsibility in them initially proved fruitless, Her responses were occasionally defensive, but more frequently were puzzled and uncomprehending.

Literal years went by before I had any sense of her early history and background. I still have remarkably little knowledge of her perceptions of her early childhood. I know that her older sister spent several years in a mental hospital. I know that she had older brothers and that her parents divorced when she was in her early teen years. Her mother remarried secretly a few years later and this was clearly a pivotal event in Sarah's life.

Gradually an image of her father emerged. He was an extremely bright and talented man, who was in school during much of her life, eventually earning a Ph.D. He was clearly the dominant figure in the family. He was occasionally physically abusive, but more frequently he controlled verbally, through sarcasm and razor-sharp intelligence. He was in many ways feared and hated. The patient recalls verbal arguments between the parents, heard while huddled in her bedroom with the other children. The sister who was hospitalized refused to allow the father even to visit her. She said she would "explain it to the patient] sometime".

To this day I have very little sense of what Sarah's mother is like. Our joint efforts to explore this area are met with a kind of fogging of the room and certainly of my own mind. If some reference is made to the mother and I attempt to clarify this, both of us become distracted. I can't remember what was said or what line of thought we were pursuing. This is also true if we are discussing her sister's hospitalization and the patient's reaction to it. Memories or events of childhood are brought out only with great difficulty. They seem to exist but cannot be readily accessed or held onto. They are also accompanied by a look in Sarah's eyes which I have come to identify as terror.

Gradually, over many years of treatment, we have become able to communicate verbally. This has come about as I have been able to abstract patterns of meaning from the fragments of largely nonverbal data which Sarah has brought in. Sometimes I was able to construct meaning from the messages on the sweatshirts she was wearing. Sometimes I could reconstruct something from her facial expressions, the presence or absence of sunglasses, or the chair in which she chose to sit. We would have conversations about the books in my bookshelves or about tiny details of my office, particularly if anything was moved. She asked me many questions about my life which I would occasionally answer briefly. It is only recently, however, that she has been able to explore the meaning behind her questions. Earlier attempts to do this were experienced by her as mystifying, rejecting, and shame-producing. I have come to understand this curiosity both about me and the details of my office as manifestations of her desire to become close to me and to my body. I believe it to be the early manifestations of a maternal erotic transference.

As a result of this early work, Sarah's communications have moved to a different developmental plane. In retrospect I believe that the work that we were doing consisted of my provision of a kind of "scaffolding" for language (Wrye and Welles, 1994) just as an attuned mother might do. A mother, for example, might say to a nine-month-old who is somewhat distressed and searching eagerly, "Oh, you're looking for your bottle," just as if the child were already able to speak. Our work together has literally provided aspects of this developmental phase which was missing in Sarah's early life.

The patient has now come to recognize that she does have inner states. These are not necessarily categorical emotions such as fear and anger, but some kind of inner experience which she is beginning to articulate verbally. The states are often quite fluid and fleeting, literally changing moment to moment. They are also very uncomfortable and distressing. She will say, "Can I leave now?" and we both understand that she is feeling uncomfortable.

As Sarah has come to realize that she does have inner experiences, she has also recognized that she isn't able to feel in the ordinary sense of the word. She has never shed a tear in my office and reported that she didn't cry when her father died. She began to be very persistent in the idea that I wasn't helping her enough, that I could do something to help her feel things. About this time and after several years of treatment, we decided to try having her on the couch, with me beside her in her peripheral vision. With hindsight I believe that this was a distancing type of maternal erotic countertransference as I attempted to pull away from her increasing demands.

While she was on the couch she began to talk more and more about her belief that I needed to help her feel things and that I could do so by touching her. If only I could touch her she would be able to feel. I began to think after all this time in treatment in which she had not even been able to a cry, this might be accomplished through physical touch. Again, looking back, I believe this was a grandiose aspect of the maternal erotic counter-transference described by Wrye and Welles (1994). Somehow I believed I could magically cure Sarah through actual contact with my body. In any case during a session on the couch she held out her hand to me and I took it.

For the next few sessions I sat in my chair beside the couch and held her hand for some part of the time. Both of us became increasingly uncomfortable. Part of my own discomfort, of course, had to do with my guilt about breaking the no touching rule of psychoanalytic treatment. But the discomfort I experienced was far greater than this. I am still uncertain as to the origin of some of the feelings but I believe they partook of fears of merger, fragmentation, engulfment, and annihilation for both of us. We mutually made the decision to stop holding hands and have not done so again.

The decision to stop at that time was ostensibly made by both of us. But in the aftermath it was as if the gates of hell were unleashed, so intense was her fury at no longer being able to do so. "Will you hold my hand?" became her battle cry, endlessly and seemingly sadistically uttered in virtually every session. Though she was often able to work productively through part of a session, as the end drew near, she would ask, plead, cajole, threaten, and then apologize and berate herself for doing so. She would ask if she were going to kill herself, would I hold her hand? This was not an idle threat given that early in treatment she had been actively suicidal. While I did not think that she would kill herself, I did have to take this comment very seriously.

As she began this intense kind of interpersonal pressure, the last five minutes of the session would seem interminable. It was as if time had stopped. She would accept none of my explanations as to why I could no longer do this. Nor could she do any exploratory work as to the meaning of these requests. This continued for many months and, at one point, she stopped treatment, feeling that she could not bring herself to stop making these requests, though at times she wanted to try.

Through consultation on the case and my own self-exploration I was finally able to understand and make use of my countertransference and thereby enable us to work through this impasse. As the grandiose omnipotent mother, I had believed I could heal Sarah through touch. Still holding onto grandiose fantasies, I now believed I could make her understand why I could not and that, through understanding, I could still meet all of her needs. Only as I was able to let go of this belief and state firmly and emphatically that I could not meet all of her needs, but I could meet some of them, were we able to move forward.

Gradually the intensity of Sarah's demands began to lessen. She became increasingly able to understand her feeling states in the session. She was able to describe several different selves who came to the sessions. One was a powerful child who totally took over. This child could not be reasoned with or controlled by other, more rational, adult selves. She also became able to view situations and people from a perspective which allows her to describe and understand what is happening.

There are still, of course, many difficult moments. In a session prior to my vacation, Sarah came in with a jumper cable wrapped around her neck. She was, however, able to identify that the powerful child was in the room and then talk about how angry the child was that I was leaving. When I told her of another upcoming vacation, she asked me to help her remember because she is aware of how angry she becomes.

In very recent weeks we have seen a new side of the child aspect of her personality. Where formerly the powerful child would appear as disruptive, angry, manipulative, even bullying, we now have access to the little Sarah who is frightened, hurt, and vulnerable. Sarah often refers to this aspect of herself in the third person, stating that she is here, but she cannot talk. The patient has also said that it is this element of her personality which holds all of her feelings. With the capability which she now has to represent her inner experience, it seems very likely that she will ultimately be able to access and integrate the feelings which have so long eluded her.

In retrospect it is perhaps inevitable that, given the intensity of this woman's longing for emotional and physical contact with me as the representation of her mother, some type of mutual enactment would occur. The fact that it occurred in the form of physical contact obviously posed special problems. It greatly intensified the transference, sometimes to unbearable levels. It further clarified for me the significance which physical contact, even as innocuous as holding hands, has for a patient. In virtually every instance of physical contact, whether it be a handshake, a pat on the shoulder or a quick hug, the meanings will be elaborated in some form or other and should ultimately be explored. The destructiveness of uncontrolled sexual contact with a patient is almost beyond imagining.

The story of Sarah illustrates many elements of the pre-representational transference. Initially, her limited capability in either understanding or expressing her experiences verbally made it necessary for us to communicate in nonverbal ways. Through data gleaned from facial expressions, body language, manner of dress, and other less readily identifiable bits of information we created a kind of nonverbal signaling which has gradually evolved into abstract symbolic form. I believe that in certain important respects I functioned as a real object for her, literally supplying the verbal scaffolding and emotional holding which, under more benign circumstances, her mother would have been able to provide. Through the enactment which occurred and Sarah's subsequent experience of my limitations and empathic failures, she has gradually been able to achieve the necessary internalization which will result in enduring structural changes.

In conclusion, the pre-representational transference emerges from a period of life which makes a rich contribution to our existence as human beings. It comes from a time when we experience life totally and globally, outside the bounds which language places upon us. As such, it is an abundant source of creativity, artistry, religion, intuition, and love. It is ours to use insofar as we are free to draw upon our early memories of those experiences within us.

To recall our experiences as infants, however, is only half of the story. The woman, the mother, who lived and shared that with us is also stored within our memories, for good or for ill. She who could enter into that world of global, body-based, sometimes chaotic, experiences, sensations, emotions, and make some sense of it for us, that woman is also within each of us. In our work with those patients who are still grounded in that nonverbal, often chaotic place, we must be able to draw upon the mother within us. Insofar as it is possible we must understand these mothering capabilities and render them explicit, conscious, and systematic. For women therapists it would entail, among other things, discussing and using unashamedly our maternal capacities. For men it may involve the exploration of fears related to regression and loss of gender identity. For all of us it will widen the scope of treatment possibilities and greatly enrich our work and our lives.

References

Bion, W.R. (1967). *Second Thoughts.* London: Karnac.

Fraiberg, S., Adelson, E. & Shapiro, V. (1975). Ghosts in the nursery: A psychoanalytic approach to the problems of impaired infant-mother relationships. *Journal of the American Academy of Child Psychiatry, 14*, 387–421.

Greenspan, S.I. (1989). *The Development of the Ego.* Madison, CT: International Universities Press, Inc.

Hirsch, M. (1989). *The Mother/Daughter Plat.* Bloomington: Indiana University Press.

Killingmo, B. (1989). Conflict and deficit: Implications for technique. *International Journal of Psychoanalysis, 70*: 65–79.

Koeple, K. (1996). Personal communication.

Krystal, H. (1988). *Integration and Self-Healing: Affect, Trauma, Alexithymia.* Hillsdale, NJ: The Analytic Press.

McDougall, J. (1989). *Theaters of the Body.* New York: Norton.

Ruddick, S, (1989). *Maternal Thinking.* Boston: Beacon Press.

Stern, D. (1985). *The Interpersonal World of the Infant.* New York: Basic Books.

Stern, D. (1995). *The Motherhood Constellation.* New York: Basic Books.

Stolorow, R. & Atwood, G. (1992). *The Intersubjective Foundations of Psychological Life.* Hillsdale, NJ: The Analytic Press.

Winnicott, D.W. (1957). *Mother and Child: A Primer of First Relationship.* New York: Basic Books.

Winnicott, D.W. (1965). *The Maturational Process and the Facilitating Environment.* New York: International Universities Press.

Wrye, H.K. & Welles, I.K. (1994). *The Narration of Desire.* Hillsdale, NJ: The Analytic Press.

Chapter Three
Clytemnestra
A Mythical Madness

From a historical perspective, the private madness of mothers is reflected and preserved in those tales that resound through the ages even as their patterns and practices continue to this day. Myth as an art form is a powerful narrator of the unconscious (Bainbridge). Authors such as Dimen, Tummala-Narra, and Joseph Campbell have clarified the ways in which these early narratives permeate the cultural unconscious so convincingly that they seem "natural" and easily codified into law. In *The Power of Myth*, Joseph Campbell describes the influential nature of myths as "the world's dreams … they are archetypal dreams and deal with great human problems" (pp. 19–20). A myth integrates an individual into society. It brings a person into harmony with the larger world. A myth is a story about a god, one who exemplifies the power and potential of a human being. Myths are neither true nor false and yet they capture the core of our humanity in metaphorical terms.

In her book *With Culture in Mind*, Muriel Dimen (2011) reinforces the influence of art and culture in its many forms upon both cultural and individual psyches. She states that "culture saturates experience. Indeed, it is the business of psychoanalysis to document this approach to treatment" (p.4). Dimen goes on to describe the concept of interpellation in which women collude in their own oppression. She argues that collusion and oppression are drawn from the same over-arching cultural

DOI: 10.4324/9781003413677-4

constructs. In her chapter in *Considering Culture from a Psychoanalytic Perspective*, Tummala-Narra (2018) reiterates this point, stating that individual psychological approaches "tend not to separate intrapsychic experience from social experience" (p.286).

It is, like art in general, a disrupter of the organized and the logical. Creative artists have, for centuries, responded to the unregulated nature of the unconscious. While psychoanalysts and academics attempt to codify it in more regulated ways, artists have long recognized the many sources of disturbance and disruption beneath the surface of life as well as the need to explore and represent them artistically. Although both art and psychoanalysis offer responses to traumatic experiences, the great artists from the Greek tragedians onward have already anticipated the unconscious landscape. As described by Bainbridge (2007), myth as an art form is a powerful narrator of the unconscious. It is, like art in general, a disrupter of the organized and the logical. Creative artists have, for centuries, responded to the unregulated nature of the unconscious. While psychoanalysts and academics attempt to codify it in more regulated ways, artists have long recognized the many sources of disturbance and disruption beneath the surface of life as well as the need to explore and represent them artistically. Although both art and psychoanalysis offer responses to traumatic experiences, the great artists from the Greek tragedians onward have preceded and anticipated the unconscious landscape.

THE ORESTEIA

The Oresteia is the focus of authors such as Rose and Jacobs. It captures the ways in which women, particularly mothers, were made to suffer. It also addresses the concept of matricide which, curiously enough, is absent from the psychoanalytic lexicon. Clytemnestra, mother of Orestes and sister of Helen of Troy, is a Spartan princess. Her first husband and their child are murdered by Agamemnon. He then rapes Clytemnestra and forces her to marry him. He orders her to produce a son and is angry and disappointed when she gives birth to three daughters—Iphigenia, Electra and Chrysothemis—before finally bearing a son, Orestes. This brutal man then kills Iphigenia as a sacrifice to ensure his victory in the Trojan War. He does so before her mother's eyes. He leaves to fight the Trojan War and returns with his mistress after ten long years whereupon Clytemnestra and her lover plot to kill him. Her son, Orestes, at the urging of Electra, later returns to the palace to avenge their father's death and kills Clytemnestra and her lover, Aegisthus.

A trial ensues and Orestes is exonerated. In an amazing twist of logic, it is reasoned that because the children do not belong to the mother, matricide is okay while patricide is not. Athena, who ostensibly has no mother, sides with Orestes who has killed his mother while Clytemnestra has committed the greater sin in killing her husband. The voices of the Furies represent the mourning that is given to women regarding their unrecognized status within the law. I am reminded of the treasured 19th century classic *Crime and Punishment* (Dostoyevsky, 2006), in which Raskolnikov brutally kills the innocent pawn broker and her sister as a way of acting out his rage against his mother. I have also observed such displacement in the dream of a client in which he attacked his beloved and elderly dog with an electric drill—a wish both phallic and murderous. Women and mothers, still disregarded, continue to haunt us with their absent presence.

Alison Stone (2012) takes issues with the idea that "the Oresteia crystallizes the overall character of ancient Greek culture" or that this "constitutes an analysis of Western civilization as a whole" (p.46). Stone argues that there have only been certain threads of matricidal thought in modern Western culture and that it is not all of modern culture that epitomizes this motif.

I believe, however, that while neither matricide nor patricide, even as expressed virtually, is visible in prevailing modern discourse, the influence of these concepts can be seen in current culture. A recent *Avenger* movie, for instance, closely parallels the perfidy of Agamemnon. The villain sacrifices his daughter to gain the favor of the gods. The stories and characters live on because they capture the fantasies, wishes, and desires that dwell outside of our awareness—mercifully repressed from their infantile state. The take-no-prisoners Agamemnon becomes a symbol of male power and aggression. This model, though infantile in its narcissism, is being acted out again and again on the current world stage.

Certainly the disregard of women and mothers, that is, their expendability, continues to exist as it did in ancient days. Mother is a constant. She is an early and enveloping presence that gives and preserves life for the human family. Her power is such that theorists such as Kristeva and Irigaray have posited that we must psychically "kill" her in order to join the symbolic universe. The semiotic nature of that original relationship has yet to be translated into the symbolic order and must, according to some theorists, be excised from consciousness as we enter the patriarchal world of language and law. In obeisance to that psychic death, these theorists have deleted women as subjects and mothers, in particular, from society in general, and, not coincidentally, from the central stage of psychoanalytic theory.

The mother-child relationship has been described as a "black hole" from which the child must disengage in order to join the symbolic universe. According to Kristeva, she or he must separate violently, that is, by means of matricide—literal or metaphoric—in order to participate in the representational world. The impact of "killing" the mother psychically is significant as will be addressed below. But when the maternal subject is invisible, submerged within the abject and the semiotic, we have no way to identify her as the focus of our study. It is furthermore difficult to recognize or evaluate the impact of matricidal wishes as long as they remain outside the bounds of symbolic discourse (Jacobs, 2007). When, however, we bring mother into the light as the object of both murderous and loving wishes and as a sentient and participating subject, we have the potential to re-evaluate the mother-child relationship. It becomes not merely a "black hole", but the repository of our deepest wishes, feelings, and dreams.

The study of mother as a participating subject also upends the patriarchal order as defined by Jacobs: "...the prototypical patriarchal myth [represents] the obliteration and appropriation of the mother's capacities in the service of the masculine project of the colonization of knowledge and generative power" (p.63). It is our focus on mother as subject, however, that can illuminate and expand our understanding of the undeniably mutual nature of the human bond.

References

Bainbridge, C. (Ed.). (2007). *Culture and the Unconscious.* New York: Palgrave Macmillan.

Campbell, J. (1988). The *Power of Myth.* New York: Doubleday.

Dimen, M. (Ed.). (2011). *With Culture in Mind.* New York: Routledge.

Dostoyevsky, F. (2006). *Crime and Punishment.* New York: Signet Classics.

Jacobs, A. (2007). *On Matricide.* New York: Columbia University Press.

Moi, T. (Ed.). (1986). *The Kristeva Reader.* Oxford: Blackwell.

Stone, A. (2012). *Feminism, Psychoanalysis and Maternal Subjectivity.* New York and London: Routledge.

Tummala-Narra, P. (2018). *Considering Culture from a Psychoanalytic Perspective.* New York: Routledge.

Whitford, M. (1991). *The Irigaray Reader.* Oxford: Blackwell.

Chapter Four
The Old Testament
Mother as Womb

The Old Testament, an arbiter of Judeo-Christian culture for thousands of years, presents its own unique challenges in efforts to unearth the story of mothers. It reiterates the idea of the maternal womb as nothing more than a breeding ground for the male sperm. We encounter pages and pages of the genealogy of the generations with no acknowledgment of the women who gave birth. In the Book of Numbers, Chapter 13, 1–16, for example, we read as follows:

> And the Lord spake unto Moses, saying, Send thou men, that they may search the land of Canaan, which I give unto the children of Israel: of every tribe of their fathers, shall ye send a man, everyone a ruler among them. And Moses by the commandment of the Lord sent them from the wilderness of Paran: all those men were heads of the children of Israel.
>
> And these were their names: of the tribe of Reuben, Shammua the son of Saccur.
>
> Of the tribe of Simeon, Shephat, the son of Hori.
>
> Of the tribe of Judah, Caleb, the son of Jeppumeh.
>
> Of the tribe of Issachar, Igal, the son of Joseph.
>
> Of the tribe of Ephraim, Oshea, the son of Nun.

DOI: 10.4324/9781003413677-5

> Of the tribe of Benjamin, Palti, the son of Raphu.
> Of the tribe of Zebulon, Gaddi, the son of Susi.
> And so forth.

In I Kings: Chapter 4, 7–19 we read as follows:

> And Solomon had twelve officers over all Israel, which provided victuals for the king and his household: each man his month in a year made provisions.
> And these are their names:
> The son of Hur, in Mount Ephraim:
> The son of Dekar, in Makaz, and in Shaalbim, and Beth-shemesh, and Elon-beth-hanan:
> The son of Hesed, in Aruboth: to him pertained Sochoh, and all the sons of Hepher:
> And so forth.

Early in the biblical narrative we encounter the stories of the powerful matriarchs. We begin with Sarah and Hagar, whose lives are intimately intertwined with each other and with Father Abraham. In Genesis 16 and 21 we read of Sarah's heartache because she cannot bear children. She carries the enormous shame that accompanies childless women in Old Testament culture. In desperation, Sarah presents Hagar to Abraham so that they may have progeny. Hagar gives birth to Ishmael and the angry and jealous Sarah insists that she be cast out into the desert. Hagar flees but is given an angelic visitation in which she is instructed to return to Abraham's home.

Sarah is also visited by God who tells her that she will have a child. She famously "laughs" because she is old and well past child-bearing years. She does, however, give birth to Isaac but she believes that Ishmael may pose a threat to her son's inheritance. She once more insists that Hagar and Ishmael be cast out. Hagar again experiences heavenly intervention and is provided with water as well as the promise that her son will be the father of nations.

The stories of Sarah and Hagar provide a compelling picture of the recurring theme of the absent presence of women in the Old Testament. Their worth—their only worth—lies in their ability to provide offspring. Perhaps they relate to their sons narcissistically, given that they represent their only avenues to vicarious power. Their presence is unmistakable but so is their absence. Where, for example, was Sarah when Abraham plans to murder their only son as a ritual sacrifice? Was she having her hair done? We simply do not know.

The abuse and subjugation of Hagar, first as a partner for Abraham—either willing or unwilling—and then as so much detritus to be cast out into the dessert carry prevailing but unspoken themes that resonate in modern society. Women may be "given" to men as a convenience—either to be raped, as spoils of war, or as the means to produce offspring—without any regard for their wishes in the matter. The ostracism of Hagar also exemplifies modern themes involving the status of Muslims and their persecution in many societies around the world.

In Genesis 27 we learn of Rebekah, the trickster. In *Women's Bible Commentary* (2012), Carol Newsom states that tricksters are a favorite vehicle for marginalized people, including foreigners, younger sons, and women, in the Old Testament. At the birth of her twin sons, Esau and Jacob, Rebekah was told by God that Jacob, who was born second, should receive the birth-rite. Since the birth-rite typically goes to the eldest son, she has to use subterfuge to ensure the birth-rite for Jacob, her favorite.

As the story goes, Isaac has grown old and blind and must confer a blessing on his eldest son before he dies. He asks Esau to hunt for game and prepare it for him to eat. Rebekah overhears the conversation and realizes that she must prepare Jacob to receive the blessing. She makes a robe for him that is hairy and reeks of the smell of the wild so that her husband will believe that it is Esau. Jacob is wary and fears that his father will discover their trickery. But he obeys his mother and thus receives his father's blessing. The ruse is successful and Jacob becomes Israel, the father of nations. Rebekah even takes the curse upon herself if they are discovered. Jacob is revered and honored throughout the Old Testament even as his mother disappears from sight. It is a familiar story of women who may gain power only through their male children.

What, we may ask, was the relationship between Rebekah and Jacob? Did she care for him as an infant or was he raised by nursemaids? Did they love one another or was he merely a "self-object" for her? Was it challenging for her to engage with Esau—perhaps a difficult "fit" between mother and child? These questions, of course, remain unanswered, but it is clear that the twins' relationship with their mother was instrumental in determining the future of the nation of Israel throughout eons of time.

In Genesis 29–31 we read of the tales of Rachel and Leah, both, in their own way, tragic heroines. Jacob meets and falls in love with the beautiful Rachel and asks her father, Laban, if he may marry her. Laban agrees but says he must first provide seven years of labor to which Jacob consents. After seven years, the wedding is arranged but Laban switches Rachel for Leah and Jacob unknowingly spends the night with the wrong woman! He must work another seven years before he can marry Rachel. Laban explains that since Leah is the older sister she must marry first.

The two women then compete over who can bear the most sons. Rachel is barren but Leah has many sons, hoping in so doing to obtain favor from Jacob. Each of the women also provide handmaidens for Jacob so that he may have even more children. Rachel finally gives birth to Joseph and Benjamin but dies in childbirth. Once again, their only worth is as the bearers of sons including Judah and Levi whose lines become critical throughout the Biblical narrative.

The two sisters are mostly obedient, their only act of rebellion occurring when they are leaving their father's house to go with Jacob. Rachel steals her father's teraphim, a statue of a minor household deity, and hides it under her saddle. Her father is outraged and searches everywhere—in the tents and packs of the caravan. When they attempt to search Rachel's belongings, she says that it is "the way of women", implying that she is menstruating. Whatever their motivations are, they leave her alone. The fact that she is menstruating renders her unclean and untouchable.

The great patriarchs make laws and fight for power against those whom God has decreed as enemies. They possess wisdom and strength that overshadow their obvious frailties. They perform miracles and are the subject of miracles. Most importantly they covenant with God; they speak with God; God speaks with them. The matriarchs provide sons to preserve a patriarchal line of descent. Once they have fulfilled their tasks relative to the bearing of children, they apparently hear no more from God and their voices too are silent.

The mothers of the Old Testament present a compelling picture of the power of women as an absent presence. They are absent in the genealogical records. They are the mothers of nations and yet their subjectivity, their personal trajectory, remains obscure. The stories of the women are significant only as they magnify the father-son relationship. We know that Sarah and Hagar were in competition for the favor of Abraham but only insofar as they gave birth to sons. Did Sarah share in the promises given to Abraham? Did she know that he was going to sacrifice Isaac? We learn nothing of Hagar's journey in the desert. Did she speak with God again? Her plight is that of single mothers throughout history—a struggle to survive.

Rachel and Leah are not the only jokesters; the only disrupters. There are others who rend the fabric of patriarchy and make decisions that are guided both by their contact with God and by their commitment to their offspring. Eve is a disrupter. She partakes of the forbidden fruit so that she and Adam can leave the garden and have children. Queen Esther, who braves the royal court and begs her husband for the lives of her people, is a disrupter. Ruth of the Old Testament is a Moabitess and a disrupter. She values intimacy and her relationship with her mother-in-law and follows her rather than conform to the patriarchal order. After the death of her husband, Ruth decides to go with Naomi. She says:

> Entreat me not to leave thee, or to return from following after thee: for whither thou goest, I will go; and where thou lodgest, I will lodge: thy people shall be my people, and thy God my God: Where thou diest, will I die, and there will I be buried: the Lord do so to me, and more also, if aught but death part thee and me.
>
> (Ruth 1:16–17.2)

I have heard the passage, set to music and sung at many weddings, but only recently have realized that the phrase is said by Ruth in reference to her mother-in-law, not her husband.

Rozmarin (2016) presents the story of Lot's wife (Genesis, 19:26) who dares to look backward to her homeland when God orders her family to leave the wicked city of Sodom. She is then turned into a pillar of salt. For Rozmarin, the mother's act of witnessing and remaining faithful to the past and acknowledging its loss is an ethical gesture that enables her daughters to create a positive genealogical relation. The mother's backward look testified to the value of life that she loved and acknowledged. She does not shut herself off from the sorrow and the loss of her life and family that has remained behind. Still, the symbol of her being turned into a pillar of salt is the ultimate in dissociation. Lot's wife is immobilized, both physically and emotionally and cannot cry out her fate!

In that sense, Lot's wife (we never know her name) is a disrupter, though the price she pays is high. We learn, for example, that two of her daughters who leave with their father decide to become impregnated by him. They apparently desire to preserve the patriarchal line which would have been broken, in that Lot would have had no sons or sons-in-law. By their actions he gains two sons who are also his grandsons. The line has been stitched up again but imperfectly so.

The women of the Old Testament are an absent presence and yet their contributions are huge—changing the trajectory of the lines of descent. They rend the fabric of patriarchy and reveal a way of life based on their own generative power. Could we not be privileged to hear their stories, their heartaches, and the private madness that could enrich our own journey as women?

References

Holy Bible, KJV. (2004). Hendrickson Bibles. Genesis 16, 21, 27, 29–31; Book of Numbers, Chapter 13, 1–16; I Kings: Chapter 4, 7–19; Numbers 13, 1–16; Ruth 1:16–17.2.

Newsome, C., Ringe, S. & Lapsley, J. (2012). *Women's Bible Commentary.* Louisville, KY: Westminster John Knox Press.

Rozmarin, M. (2016). Staying Alive: Matricide and the Ethical-political Aspects of Mother-Daughter Relations. *Studies in Gender and Sexuality*, *17*(40), 242–253.

Chapter Five
Old Testament Remnants in Psychoanalysis

Turning now to the 20th century, we encounter the myriad ways in which the status of women and mothers remains basically unchanged. We may or may not be familiar with the Old Testament but its influence on traditional psychoanalysis is undeniable. While Freud described himself as "completely estranged" from Judaism, he remained essentially Jewish. He seemed not fully aware of his Jewish "character", thus lending it a mystical quality which remained unexplored and largely unconscious. One may speculate that it stemmed from his identification with his mother who was well versed in Jewish tradition and theology.

For my argument, I will consider four concepts from the Old Testament that are replicated in psychoanalysis as they preserve and continue the absence of women and mothers. These omissions are observable within the following constructs: biblical narrative; structure over sensuality; the male body as the prototype; and compassion versus appropriation.

BIBLICAL NARRATIVE

The father-son relationship is the seminal narrative both in the Biblical account and in Freud's psychoanalysis. The Biblical story of Jacob, the Jewish patriarch, is replicated in the Oedipus myth which is, in turn, the organizing relationship within traditional psychoanalysis. Jacob was not

DOI: 10.4324/9781003413677-6

the favorite of his father and, though he did not strive to kill his father, he did not hesitate to trick him at the urging of his mother. In fact, as with Freud, Jacob was the favorite of his mother. Though he was the second of the twin sons, his mother had received a revelation that he was to have the birthright. Jacob was apparently clutching the heel of his brother, Esau, as they emerged from the womb.

As in traditional psychoanalysis, the role of the mother is minimized. Rebekah's presence is given scant reference even though she is central to the story. God spoke to her and let her know that her second son, Jacob, was to receive the birth right. She was the prime mover in an act that would reverberate throughout the Biblical narrative. Nevertheless, she is seldom seen as anyone of importance. As with psychoanalytic theory, she is a support person or an object of desire. She is a daughter, a mother, a wife and her importance is as a bearer of male children and as a link to the generations.

STRUCTURE OVER PERSONAL

An Old Testament theme that is also reflected in Freud's version of psychoanalysis is the predominance of structure over the personal and the individual. The Biblical account changes from the personal conversations with God to a structured and hierarchical obeisance to authority. In Genesis, for example, God speaks directly to Abraham, Sarah, Rebecca, and others. By the time God interacts with Moses, however, the communication takes place through signs and symbols, such as a burning bush. Over time, religion becomes enclosed in signs and symbols. A hierarchy of authority is in place with priests and rabbis designated as intermediaries. It becomes a patriarchal structure in which those who are called may see and hear him while those who are not so authorized may discern him only through a specified hierarchy.

Again, Freud replicates this development. In *Moses and Monotheism*, he places the patriarchal structure over that of a matriarchal society. He acknowledges that matrilineal societies had existed in the past but that, in the course of history, matriarchy was succeeded by patriarchy. As Sprengnether (1990) points out, his argument is convoluted and struggles to account for powerful female deities. It does, however, enshrine a patriarchal and structured religion with its accompanying signs and symbols over a matriarchal and personalized relationship with deity. Thus, as with the religion of old, it minimizes the significance of women and mothers for whom direct personal communication is essential. The relationship between Yahweh and Jacob—illustrating the tension between father and son—evolves into a formal structure of male priests and laymen. Jewish women could take pride in the lofty nature of their sons' positions but were excluded from reading the Torah. The turning from the mother to the father denotes a triumph of the hierarchical over the sensual and the personal. It is considered an advance in culture in which the maternal configuration, relying on the quality of the senses, is deemed inferior to the paternal structure that rests on logical premise and conclusion.

CASTRATION, CIRCUMCISION AND THE MALE BODY AS PROTOTYPE

A third construct that illustrates the influence of the Old Testament upon psychoanalysis is reflected in the focus on the male body as the prototype. Circumcision, as the mark of the Abrahamic covenant, valorizes the male body and thus provides a link to Father Abraham and the blessings and promises which he can provide. In Genesis 12: 2–3 God covenants with Abraham, stating that he will bless him and his seed and make of him a great nation and that in him all families of the earth will be blessed. The sign of the covenant of the chosen people was circumcision. The matriarchs whose pregnant bodies generate that posterity are not mentioned for their contributions.

Freud's focus was also on the male body. He regarded circumcision as a symbolic token of castration which facilitated both the advance to a world of abstract rules and concepts and the renunciation of the sensual and the magical. The commandments and covenants, the prohibition against idols, and the internalization of an abstract, invisible divine spirit representing ethical perfection "forced upon the people an advance in intellectuality which, important enough in itself, opened the way, in addition, to the appreciation of intellectual work and to further renunciations of instinct" (p.123). God's message to Moses, as portrayed by a burning bush, valorized an invisible deity who demanded a life of truth and justice and exacted vengeance on those who did not comply.

Thus women and their pregnant bodies are absent from the Old Testament and the psychoanalytic equivalent. In the Bible they are mentioned as "wombs" and, in psychoanalytic theory, their pregnant bodies are described as compensation for the lack of a penis. If the ego is a body ego, it follows that a woman would be invested in a body that allows her to bear children if she so chooses. But traditional theory would have her mourn for a part of the anatomy that she never had. Her real experience would remain in a pre-verbal world of illusion, one which must be forgotten in order to enter the patriarchal structure.

COMPASSION VERSUS APPROPRIATION

The Old Testament contributions to Freud's view of human nature are striking. In Genesis, chapter 22, we read of Abraham's willingness to sacrifice his son as a burnt offering as well as Isaac's acquiescence. There is no mention either of the trauma that Isaac would have felt or of the presence of Sarah. Did she know? If so, did she agree? From a modern perspective or *any* perspective it is difficult to imagine that a mother would agree to the sacrifice of her only son.

Isaac grows up and marries Rebekah and the trend continues. Rebekah is regarded as devious, a trickster, and she is. But she also communes with God who tells her that her second son Jacob is to have the birthright. How does she navigate her lack of power in a patriarchal society given the inspiration she believes to have come from God? Is she afraid? Does she fear for her son's well-being? Her own? She is powerful but she does not have direct access to power. Like Hagar, she appears to be mindful only of the welfare of her son.

The Old Testament is clearly not an account that records feeling and emotion. The violent narratives are stated matter-of-factly and without attention to the sentiments that would certainly have occurred. It is likely however that they would have affected men and women differently. Men were in the center of battle and were routinely slaughtered at the whim of male leaders who were apparently directed by God. Women were at the margins—trying to protect their children—with bare mention of their efforts, their fears, their loves, or their communication with deity.

The Biblical tales of appropriation, as evidenced in battles, rapes, and endless slaughter and presented as righteous obliteration countenanced by God, are reiterated in the work of Hobbes, Nietzsche, and Freud. A classical psychoanalytic account of human nature describes acquisitive creatures who must sacrifice needs and wants in order to live together. In *Compassion, Dialogue, and Context: On Understanding the Other* by Roger Frie, Ph.D. and Psy.D., the authors state that revisionist psychoanalysts may overlook Freud's negative and pessimistic view of human nature. Frie pointed out the traditionl psychoanalytic view of the "other" as reflected in a quote from Nietzsche, of whom Freud was a devoted follower:

> Life itself is essentially appropriation … [it is] injury, overpowering of the alien and weak, oppression, hardness, imposition of form, incorporation and, at the very least—gain. … Appropriation does not simply belong to a perverse or imperfect or primitive society: it belongs in essence to living things, as an organic basic function.
>
> (p.259)

Sprengnether points out that Freud continues this trend. In his description of the dream of Irma's injection, he "dissociates himself from Irma as a victim of physical violation in order to confirm himself in the less threatening, if professionally problematic, role of her physician" (p.171). Irma's subjective experience is not addressed in the course of her treatment. As in Biblical times, he does not address the emotional toil which, Irma, would have undoubtedly suffered.

Freud's own account of his interaction with his father in the "Hat in the Gutter Story" conveys his commitment to appropriation and vengeance. He states as follows:

> It was on one such occasion, that he told me a story to show me how much better things were now than they had been in his day. "When I was a young man," he said, "I went for a walk one Saturday;… I was well dressed, and had a new fur cap on my head. A Christian came up to me and with a single blow knocked off my cap into the mud and shouted: 'Jew! Get off the pavement!'" "And what did you do?" I asked. "I went into the roadway and picked up my cap," was his quiet reply. This struck me as unheroic conduct on the part of the big, strong man who was holding the little boy by the hand. I contrasted this situation with another which fitted my feelings better: the scene in which Hannibal's father … made his boy swear before the household altar to take vengeance on the Romans.
>
> (Freud, 1900, p. 197)

References

Blatt, D. (1988). The Development of the Hero: Sigmund Freud and the Reformation of the Jewish Tradition. *Psychoanalysis and Contemporary Thought*, *11*(4), 639–703.

Blum, H.P. (1991). Freud and the Figure of Moses: The Moses of Freud. J. Amer. *Psychoanalytic Association*, *39*: 513–535.
Freud, S. (1939). Moses and monotheism. 3–137.
Frie, R. Ph.D. *Compassion, Dialogue, and Context: On Understanding the Other.*
Holy Bible, KJV. (2019). Christian Art Publishers, Genesis 12: 2–3.
Sprengnether, M. (1990). *The Spectral Mother.* Ithaca, NY: Cornell University.

Chapter Six
Quilters
Remnants of Women's Lives

In *Woman: A Global Chronicle of Gender Inequality*, Nina Ansary states that women in general have historically been without a voice, without recognition. She quotes Virginia Woolf, who concluded: "Indeed, I would venture to guess that ANON, who wrote so many poems without signing them, was often a woman" (p.1). Ansary states that women in general have for the last 4000 years had to remain invisible because of the restrictions placed on their gender. She then chronicles the extraordinary accomplishments of the women of history—great innovators who have remained unknown despite their contributions to every aspect of life, that is, scientific, literary, medical, political, that we take for granted. All of her examples were born before 1900 and date back to 2300 BCE.

An early example Ansary provides is that of Cleopatra Metrodora who lived around 200–400 CE. She was a Greek physician and her work is considered to be the first medical treatise written by a woman. She, of course, studied the female body and those diseases particular to women. She was able to ascertain the presence of sexual abuse, cure local infections, perform cosmetic breast and facial reconstruction, and recommend surgical treatment for breast and uterine cancer. But, as with other women innovators, her work remained unknown for many centuries.

In a story much like that of Clytemnestra, Gaitana was a 16th century woman in Columbia who organized 6000 Yalcon people to rebel against

DOI: 10.4324/9781003413677-7

the Spanish conquistador Pedro de Anasco. It is believed that Gaitana disrespected the orders of Anasco who then burned her son alive in her presence. Gaitana sought revenge and captured Anasco and his men. As a punishment she tore his eyes out and dragged him by a noose until he died. Her unspeakable act matched the brutality of her oppressor but, nevertheless, her astonishing courage has finally been recognized with a sculpture created in 1974 by Rodrigo Arenas Betancourt that depicts a female Yalcon warrior known to be Gaitana.

My favorite example is that of Lillian Gilbreth, who was a 20th century pioneer of industrial and organizational psychology. She was also the mother of 12 children and their fame is immortalized in the movie the *Cheaper By the Dozen*. She and her husband wrote a number of books but her name was always excluded because it was assumed that a woman listed as an author would detract from the books' credibility. After her husband's untimely death she continued her work and set up training workshops for those who wanted to apply the principles of industrial psychology that they had learned. The workshops were held in her home so that she could supervise the children while she worked. She may have been the first 20th century woman to "have it all".

These women visionaries, warriors, diplomats, and scientists remained anonymous until Ansary and others pursued their stories. That half of the population had to work in silence and in secret because of the heavy gender restrictions of their day, some of which have continued into the present. It is likely that most of them were mothers and, if so, their astonishing contributions would have been created in and around the daily work of mothering. Like their creative endeavors, their tasks as mothers would have remained invisible, even to them.

We see that these women, these innovators who were also very likely mothers, were either unbelievably powerful or invisible. The tales of Gaitana or Clytemnestra murdering the brutal men who killed their children strike fear in our hearts. The day-to-day accounts of Gilbreth as the mother of 12 children are yet unknown. We have no lasting narratives of the quotidian experiences and fantasies of mothers who have raised the world's children. We have but minimal accounts on gravestones or funeral urns or in the pages of diaries that have been miraculously preserved.

We may occasionally encounter art forms that depict the mother experience in stories, pictures, and songs without words. The quilters of 19th century America have attempted to record their narratives in the beautiful quilts they made. Their efforts were born of necessity and quilting as an art form provided a means of expression otherwise unavailable to them. The quilts were made out of rags, or small pieces of cloth from which the women could piece together exquisite patterns of shape and color. They had names like Log Cabin, Diamond Field, Lone Star, and Tree of Life and the patterns and topics often mirrored the seminal events in their lives. A Double Wedding Ring would, of course, coincide with a wedding and a Star of Bethlehem, a Christmas theme.

The quilts also depicted the dark side of life—the deaths and losses; the miscarriages and the abortions. Such events were illustrated by means of "shadow blocks": shadow blocks were not always tragic but were used to evoke the unspoken fears as well as the presence of mystery and death (Newman and Damashek, 1986).

In their book *The Quilters: Women and Domestic Art: An Oral History* (Cooper and Allen, 1999), the authors completed extensive interviews with a group of women quilters in Texas and New Mexico. They learned that the quilts and the preparations for them were expressions of the women's lives. A woman named Mary recounts the hardships over which they have no control—a hail storm, a bad crop, a prairie fire. The quilting—the piecing together of scraps of material—allows her to bring together the fragments of her life and thus create order through her art.

The circumstances of their lives are heart-wrenching and often tragic. The play *Quilters*, for example, also brings to life a scene called Secret Drawer. Mabel Louise writes to her sister Harriet to tell her that she is expecting her 12th child that winter. She begs the doctor for help to terminate the pregnancy, explaining that she is 35 and that if she dies there will be no one to care for her husband and her children. The doctor knows what she is asking and, of course, refuses her request. Mabel Louise's sister sends her a recipe that she believes will help. It consists of klipsweet and pennyroyal; a cup of quinine and a handful of human hair and she is to drink the whole concoction down at once. When swallowed it will bring about stomach contractions. Though far away Harriet sends her loving thoughts and prayers to her sister.

As the drama unfolds, a chorus, much like the Greek chorus of ancient times, intones the names of the children born and miscarried. A 12th child Ellie is born and miscarried. A 13th named Alan is also miscarried. Luke is a 15th child, dead at birth. The litany of names attests to the heartache of unwanted pregnancies and lack of any access to reliable birth control.

In the context of this discussion, it becomes clear that the lives of these women who were mothers were represented in remnants, rags, and discarded fragments of fabric from which they attempted to piece together the history of their lives, their communities and their family ties. Like the quilts, their lives were tattered, interrupted again and again by the movement of their households, the losses they endured, the endless back-breaking physical work, and the loneliness of the plains and prairies. There was no continuous thread of accomplishment, no monuments to their efforts, and no accounts in the history books, no towns and cities named in their honor. Yet the ten or eleven children that they bore and struggled to raise to adulthood populated the American West.

Who were these women, these mothers of nations? Some were great artists as exemplified in the colors and patterns of their magnificent quilts, only some of which are preserved. They were humanitarians—helping and succoring one another—in childbirth, sickness, and death. They were prairie doctors—learning of herbal remedies and procedures they could employ when "real" doctors were unavailable. They were marksmen—learning to shoot marauders and wild game for food when their husbands were absent or dead. All of these responsibilities were in addition to their "womanly" duties of housekeeping and childcare. The quilts they made were a means of expression, a way of preserving their existence for ensuing generations.

It is true that the stories of the men of the prairies are also unknown but they had their heroes—sheriffs and gunslingers, governors, generals, good men who were their obvious roles models and who could provide codes of conduct for them to emulate. Women's lives were lived in private and in secret, known only to mothers and sisters, and never rising to the level of protagonist within the pioneer story. The opportunity to write and preserve a cohesive history—a profoundly human enterprise—was rarely available to them. Yet they persevered and rendered from snippets of cloth the fragments of their tattered lives. Their stories provide a visual representation of the fragmented and interrupted inner world that many women experience.

References

Ansary, N. (2020a). *Anonymous is a Woman*. Revela Press.

Ansary, N. (2020b). *Woman: A Global Chronicle of Gender Inequality.* Los Angeles, CA: Revela Press.

Cooper, P.J. & Allen, N.B. (1999). *The Quilters: Women and Domestic Art: An Oral History.* Lubbock, TX: Texas Tech. University Press.

Newman, M. and Damashek, B. (1986). *Quilters.* Lubbock, TX: Texas Tech. University Press.

Chapter Seven
Relational Theory and the "Absent Presence"

Jacobs (2007) points out that the symbolic order has excluded the subjective maternal and has foreclosed a symbolically mediated mother-daughter relationship. The emergence of a relational developmental model of human growth has however shifted our focus to the period of life before symbolic representation becomes primary. Joyce McDougall states that "…our classical psychoanalytic models of mental functioning, to the extent that they are based on meaning, are insufficient for conceptualization of the manner in which psychic life is organized from the period before the infant becomes a verbal child…" (1989, p.36). She continues:

> What has emerged from our greatly increased understanding of this early phase of life is a realization of the extraordinary complexity of the mother/infant relationship. Though the communication is largely non-verbal, certainly on the part of the infant, mother and child are found to be engaging in a complex continuing social dialogue, one which is absolutely crucial in the formation of a human being.
>
> (1999, p.37)

DOI: 10.4324/9781003413677-8

Daniel Stern's pioneering work (1995) has, for example, endeavored to identify and clarify the nature of the early mother-child relationship through the painstaking study of the hundreds of daily, minute-by-minute, nonverbal interactions that comprise their life together. The mother's effective participation depends on her ability to read and empathize with the baby's nonverbal cues. His focus is, however, on the mother only as she interacts with her child. There is little recognition of her status as a person with an identity other than "mother".

In fact, current influential research has promulgated the idea that the child must find only herself in the mind of mother. Peter Fonagy (2002) describes a process that he calls "markedness" in which the mother may replicate the child's emotion but must show no "real" emotion of her own. To do so would dysregulate the child, that is, overwhelm her with more than she could process. Winnicott states that the infant needs to find himself in the mother's mind, not the mother herself (1965). The point of this and other texts that describe optimal conditions for the baby is that they indicate that the mother's needs must in no way impinge upon the infant. Her task, her only task, is that of mirroring and tuning in with the required amount of empathic attention and emotional engagement. This type of self-effacement would be a challenge for even the most experienced clinician within a traditional psychoanalytic paradigm. We can recognize that the mother's emotion may be too much for a child to bear on an ongoing basis, but we must find a way to yet recognize her subjective feelings and experience.

We cannot as yet contemplate the "mind of mother". Stern (1995) has pointed out that mother's experience has existed largely outside of consciousness, not only for the mother, but for everyone. In the years of our infancy, this being has untold power, and it is her will and her ministrations that keep us alive. She herself seems unable even to begin to describe what she is doing, what it feels like, and how she accomplishes it. It has remained in that realm of human experience occupied by the poetic, the spiritual, and the mystical. Mother as a reactive three-dimensional human being—at best, distractible, preoccupied, overwhelmed, and exhausted, and at worst, frightened, ill, hungry, over-worked, and alone—has very little place either in history or culture.

The pre-verbal mother-child relationship is just that—nonverbal. The mother and baby are in close physical proximity. As described by Wrye and Wells:

> The infant, having once been literally encapsulated in mother's womb in amniotic fluid, experiences closeness postnatally through contact with skin and bodily fluids, through her caretaking in relation to milk, drool, urine, feces, mucus, spit, tears, and perspiration. A mother's contact with and ministrations to her baby in dealings with these fluids may optimally create a slippery, sticky sensual adhesion in the relationship; it is, so to speak, the medium for bonding. This sensuality, experienced by both parties, is key in their relationship.
>
> (1994, p.35)

In my own experience of mothering, I was astounded, gob-smacked, by the *fluids* which enveloped the experience. In the early days, I encountered blood that resulted from an emergency C-section. As the weeks went, by I confronted leaking milk, urine, feces, tears (my own), and other unidentifiable substances that left both baby and mother feeling soaked and wet on a continuing basis.

It is this non-verbal, chaotic, and yet intensely sensual and pleasurable, experience that we need to "kill" even as we long for its return. It is a time before language and we acknowledge it at our peril in a world that valorizes the verbal, the representational, the logical, and the organized over that which we cannot begin to describe. To acknowledge consciously mother's biological capabilities and her psychological presence would be to validate her enormous power. To view mother as an individual means that we disentangle our deeply-held beliefs from the complex interweaving of biology and male dominance that has held us captive. We would then be compelled to consider different and disturbing data that have seldom entered our conscious minds. It would be terrifying to contemplate the concept of mother, the shadowy presence that, for good or ill, infuses all of our lives, as anything other than an always-available but largely invisible, primal energy. It would open us to a recognition, not only of mother's generative power—literally over life and death—but also to the memories of untold joy, mutual adoration, and well-being for which we long.

References

Benjamin, J. (1988). *The Bonds of Love. Psychoanalysis, Feminism and the Problem of Domination*. New York: Pantheon Books.

Fonagy, P. (Ed.). (2002). *Affect Regulation, Mentalization and the Development of the Self.* New York: Other Press.
Jacobs, A. (2007). *On Matricide: Myth, Psychoanalysis, and the Law of the Mother.* New York: Columbia University Press.
McDougall, J. (1985). *Theatres of the Body.* New York: Routledge.
Mitchell, S. and Aron, L. (1991). *Relational Psychoanalysis and the Emergence of a Tradition.* Hillsdale, NJ: The Analytic Press.
Stern, D. (1995). *The Motherhood Constellation.* New York: Basic Books.
Winnicott, D.W. (1965). *The Naturational Process and the Facilitating Environment.* London: Routledge.
Wrye, H.K. and Wells, I.K. (n.d.) *The Narration of Desire.* Hillsdale, NJ: The Analytic Press.

CHAPTER EIGHT
THE MATERNAL BODY IN PSYCHOANALYSIS

In both the Old and New Testament, the maternal body has been referred to as a "womb" from which important men emerge. God communicates with the woman in whose womb the men are housed so that she is informed as to their importance. He has little to say to her throughout the remaining narrative. He seldom interacts with the living woman who is going to give birth. At this late stage in human history can we yet extract a plausible narrative for the maternal body and, most especially, the woman herself?

Balsam discusses Daniel Stern's view in *The Motherhood Constellation* in which he proposes a new mental state in which the mother is able to focus completely on her child. He does not address, however, the idea that she is still a sexual being, a separate being with her own identity, her own thoughts and fantasies which are not focused on her child. In that regard, a child would find in the so-called "mind of the mother" something other than a preoccupation with him.

The ego is a body ego and, according to Balsam, the castration complex would be cogent for males but not for females because it is not based on female anatomy. The lack of attention to the pregnant female body has continued with a few exceptions which have not been integrated into mainstream theory or practice. Balsam cites the concept of "female genital anxiety", which may encompass the woman's experience

DOI: 10.4324/9781003413677-9

regarding her own internal organs which can miraculously create a baby. The author further cites the postmodern influence in which the body is a mental construct. Postmodern theory has allowed us to rethink gendered power relations and embrace multiple sexual identities but it once again ignores the female body and its procreative abilities.

Other modern attempts to reclaim female anatomy are addressed by Holtsman and Kulish (2000) in their article "Nevermore: The Hymen and the Loss of Virginity". The authors explore the meaning of the hymen in myth, literature, and clinical work. They suggest that both male and female anatomy have bisexual components—the foreskin representing the female aspect in the man and the hymen, the male aspect in the woman. The authors state that their patients indicated an unconscious connection between the foreskin and the hymen which thus fosters the mutual identification that may occur during defloration.

Jill Salberg 2007claims that Freud's attention to the navel is the closest he comes to acknowledging true mystery and she ties it to an unconscious recognition of femininity, the body, and the mother. She notes that he focuses on the navel in a recorded dream as it connects to the maternal. Jay Eatson also refers to the "navel" of psychic development as an identification with the mother. It is "unknown" to him not because it is unknowable but because he is a man. Manhood in a patriarchal culture depends on denying, in myriad ways, the powerful ambivalence that the mother inspires. Thus rather than felling, condemning, or idealizing the body of the (m)other, we need to recognize her in ourselves.

Balsam has further opened the discussion of female anatomy and has paved the way for us to consider the impact of pregnancy on a woman's subjective experience. She considers the concept of plasticity, in which a woman's body changes shape so as to accommodate another human. With this, I would include the idea of permeability. A woman carries another being within her for nine months and her body boundaries are thus compromised. We can assume that her psychic boundaries are also permeable—a phenomenon that may be connected to the so-called "borderline" personality disorder. Her body has been intruded upon by a "little stranger". Add to this the frequent and often unwelcome commentary made by total strangers who may guess the due date, size, and weight of the baby as a woman nears term. This intrusion, both internal and external, is in addition to the current government intrusion into the pregnant woman's body.

A woman's relationship to her child and vice-versa is never free from the original merging of bodies. It is not imaginary but rather a physical oneness in which the fetus is quite literally dependent on the "host", the mother for nutrients, water—life itself. The first three months of life are considered by many to be an external womb… a kangaroo pouch?

I gave birth to my four sons in the seventies and eighties. It was popular at that time to write birthing experiences and I did so for all of my pregnancies. The first birthing was a 24-hour labor and, in as much as the labor was progressing slowly, there was the possibility that I might need a C-section. I was dehydrated and exhausted. The baby was "sunny side up" and after the head was turned, the doctor instructed me to push. My husband reported that my strength was "off the charts". My own experience was that *I was God*, the creator of the universe.

The middle deliveries were long (eight hours each) but, in comparison, relatively unremarkable. My fourth delivery progressed slowly and finally came to a standstill. My doctor, who to my knowledge remained childless, noted that the fetal heartbeat had become erratic. She decided that I must have an emergency C-section. I am relatively immune to anesthetic so I still felt the cutting. My son was gorgeous and healthy and weighed in at 9 pounds and 2 ounces. I remembered very little but months later I had a traumatic flashback of being cut into along with the searing pain that it entailed.

My point is that pregnancy is not always a walk in the park. The experiences of birthing are tough to remember because the mind and body mercifully blot them out in short hours after birth. It seems to be essential so that the species can go forward. I recall an incident some years later when we were at an amusement park where I reluctantly agreed to ride the Iron Dragon. It is an enclosed roller coaster with many dips, twists, and turns and I was clinging to some other human for dear life. Afterward my boys asked me what it felt like. I said it felt like a birth canal. They laughed uproariously. They have grown accustomed to having an analyst for a mother. But that is what it felt like to me—utterly terrifying both for the child being born and for the mother who does the birthing.

The psychic consequences of the birthing experiences for both mother and child have focused largely on the child. The mother's experience of literally holding a being inside her body and then subsequently being able to separate has, to my knowledge, not been considered. Yet the woman's ability or lack thereof to separate has been the stuff of scorn and disparagement. Can we begin to address the ways in which she manages that transition? Can we even consider it from her perspective? Is it holding? Embracing? Suffocating? What about the movement of the fetus? What meaning does that have *for the mother*? I know my own experience has been a sense of mourning and loss once the birth occurs. *I missed my constant little companion. I felt lonely.* Are those feelings aberrant? The experiences of a neurotic clinging mother from whom the child must forcibly eject? What if they are okay? What if they are the beginnings of a lifelong relationship from the mother's perspective? The biological and psychological experiences of holding and creating life are Godlike in their significance. Can we not then find them a place in psychoanalytic theories that purport to describe life in its very depths?

References

Balsam, R. (2012). *Women's Bodies in Psychoanalysis.* New York and London: Routledge.

Eatson, J. (1995). Guys and Dolls: Exploratory Repetition and Maternal Subjectivity in the Fort/Da Game. *American Imago*, *52*(4), 463–503.

Holtsman, D. and Kulish, N. (2000) *Nevermore: The Hymen and the Loss of Virginity.* Northvale, NJ: Aronson.

Salberg, J. (2007). The Vanishing Mother: Reply to Commentaries. *Psychoanal. Dial.*, *17*(2): 239–245.

Chapter Nine
A Theory of Matricide

The law of the mother lies hidden, as Jacob Arlow (1982) expressed, behind the screen of unconscious fantasies. It is an arena that is both too tender and too horrific to contemplate. Its acknowledgment would bring into conscious awareness our vital dependence on our mothers and our reliance on their procreative powers in the preservation of the species. Within the order of language and symbolic representation, it is the law of the father that currently presides. It is the arbiter in major corporate entities; the political arena; the doctrines of world religions; warfare; and Wall Street. Women's contribution merits a footnote in our cultural history but her subjective presence remains anonymous. As Ansary points out in her compendium of influential but unrecognized women of history, whenever an invention, a work of art, or a piece of music is considered "anonymous," it is most likely the creation of a woman. (*Anonymous is a Woman.*) She is lost to the dust of the ages and to our own murky preverbal past.

Maternal subjectivity is a difficult landscape without the usual verbal markers of language. How do we explore the non-verbal when the symbolic world of language is dominant? Jacobs states that there is not a real mother but merely a theoretical concept as Lacan would have it. Do we leave it at that—mother in the realm of the imaginary? What about the very real existence that mothers inhabit as they care

DOI: 10.4324/9781003413677-10

for the young? How do we enter the debates on mothering practices, postnatal depression, child-rearing practices; mothering and work; breast feeding and the like? How do we figure out just what a mother is doing as she cares for an infant, attends to a two-year-old tugging at her shirt, arranges a carpool for soccer practice, and tries to imagine dinner for a family of five? It is my intention to address both the theory and practice of mothering in a manner that brings her reality into existence.

Curiously enough, the concept of matricide recognizes mother as an agent of meaning. An early article by R. M. Linder (1948) lists the ways in which matricide can be acted out, including actual murder and suicide. He cites the ways in which it has been psychically converted as in acting out, dreams, displacement, reaction formation, and repression. He describes its appearance in schizophrenia in which the wish may be verbalized even while it remains hidden in neurotic patients. The author also states that many analyses fail because the matricidal impulse is so overlaid with defenses and disguises as to make it impossible to discover.

Both Kristeva (1989) and Irigaray (1985) have brought into our awareness the absence of a concept of theoretical matricide, given the lack of awareness of mothers as subjects. They have also deemed matricide as a necessity in order to enter the symbolic and patriarchal universe. They view it as a function of the need to distance from the maternal body; to "kill" the mother of infancy. The injunction is stated by Kristeva as follows: "For man and for woman the loss of the mother is a biological and psychic necessity, the first step on the way to autonomy. Matricide is our vital necessity, the sine qua non of our individuation" (p. 38).

They also point out that theoretical matricide exacts a price in that the child loses the corporeal and emotional connection to the mother. Kristeva, for instance, discusses the etiology of depression in women. In addition to the more frequently cited factors such as hormonal imbalance and the denigration of female experience, she includes the devastating loss of the early connection to the maternal body. According to Kristeva, the body's semiosis must become lost or repressed in order for women and men to enter the world of language, meaning, and logic. Yet the resulting symbolic representation of mother and child may seem distant and "false".

The position of Luce Irigaray states that in Western culture the child must break from the maternal body and the early relationship in order to join the symbolic order. It becomes a difficult choice for the girl child in particular, in that she must break from her mother in order to partake of the symbolic and yet identify with her in order to assume a female identity. The female must negate the tie with the mother and rediscover her through distant representation. Irigaray insists that patriarchal culture or cultures need to change in directions that would permit daughters to differentiate themselves psychically from their mothers.

Patriarchal texts do give credence to the early mother-child bond, but, like these early theorists, view it as a tie which may be broken with little recognition of the tragic consequences. Returning once more to the biblical account of Lot's wife, Sheehy (2012) notes that her story actually valorizes women's silence, showing that they suffer from fear of challenging the prevailing discourse; fear of being judged or written off; fear of speech itself. It is, in my view, a bit of a twist to see the fate of Lot's wife as anything other than the tragic consequence of a vengeful God who has no truck with disobedience even if it is merely a woman who wishes to remain connected with her home and family. It has taken 5000 years to recognize the significance of her role as witness and connecter.

Sheehy also points to the New Testament story of the Virgin Mary, a seminal figure in Christian theology. Mary is subjected to paternal law and becomes at best an instrument that brings about the birth of Jesus. Mary's experience of being the mother of Christ is encapsulated all too briefly in the phrase "she kept all these things and pondered them in her heart" (Luke 2–19). She does not appear again until the Crucifixion. As Kristeva points out (1987), the maternal body is venerated, as is the Virgin Mary, but also denigrated as abject, a site of horror, disgust, and revulsion.

Stone (2016) also cites the difficulty of extracting women's positive experience from patriarchal accounts. The position of Lot's wife is clearly fixed by patriarchy. We learn that Lot is a righteous man who is warned by God to leave the wicked city of Sodom. (Genesis 19:26) Lot's wife (we never learn her name) commits the "sin" of disobeying God by looking back both to the city she loves and the plight of her two daughters who remain there. The moral of the story illustrates the power of God's wrath and the danger of "looking back" to remember ties of love and connection—"maternal ties".

Stone takes issue with the "seeds of hope" as proposed by Rozmarin in that Lot's wife dies and thus the surviving daughters have no way of retaining a loving relationship with her except in memory. She contends that we have to re-weave a positive relationship with our mothers—one that we recognize and one that has an acknowledged place within our culture. She states as follows:

> In re-reading and tarrying with the patriarchal past, then, we come full circle and remember Lot's wife. We do so by re-enacting her gesture: that of looking backward, remaining connected to our backgrounds and resisting the symbolic law that commands us to break from those backgrounds absolutely.
>
> (2016, p.260)

Amber Jacobs states that since there is no place in psychoanalytic theory for a maternal subject, the law of the father encompasses all symbolization. Her focus is one of creating the law of the mother by bringing the mother-child relationship into the symbolic order. At present, the symbolic order excludes the subjective maternal and forecloses a symbolically mediated mother-daughter relationship. To address that omission, Jacobs draws from Greek myth in order to build a theory that recognizes the maternal subject and thus brings matricide into representational discourse.

Again, it is the Orestia myth as recounted by Jacobs that provides insight into what she regards as a universal matricidal phantasy. A primal phantasy is regarded as being a universal structure, but at present the maternal subject is, as Jacobs points out, restricted and excluded. Metis, the first wife of Zeus, wanted to escape his advances and thus changed into all different forms. She was caught by Zeus and impregnated. Before she gave birth, she was swallowed whole by him. From his belly Metis advised Zeus and gave him her wisdom. A few months later he felt a terrible pain in his head which finally split open, revealing Athena. Metis was never heard from again.

Zeus cannibalizes Metis in order to gain both her wisdom and knowledge and her procreative power. It consolidates and maintains a paternal law that depends on the eradication of that power. This theme is repeated in the Old Testament, in which women are talked about in regard to birthing but then never heard from again. In the trial that exonerates Orestes for the crime of matricide, Athena defends him by saying that she herself had no mother (born as she was from the head of her father Zeus), but in fact she did. In recognizing the absent mother of Athena who was incorporated by her husband, Jacobs illustrates that matricide is, in fact, a universal phantasy that precedes patricide. As we "keep hold" of Metis, we acknowledge the law of the mother, embodied in the life-giving potential of women. Thus we recognize its political significance as it both illuminates and defends against the envy men have of women's real generative power.

We can then gaze beneath the secure and even sacred umbrella which patriarchy provides and observe motives which are all too human. Mary O'Brien declares that patriarchy grows out of men's efforts to ensure historical continuity in the absence of biological continuity (2007). She writes as follows: "Paternity, then, is not a natural relationship to a child, but a right to a child … It is the historical movement to provide this support system which transforms the individual uncertainties of paternity into the triumphant universality of patriarchy" (p.75). It is maternal subjectivity that can loosen and re-align its grip.

References

Arlow, J. (1982). Scientific Forum.

Ansary, N. (2020). *Anonymous is a Woman*. Revela Press.

Dostoyevsky, F. (2001). *Crime and Punishment* (C. Garnett, Trans.). Mineola, NY: Cornell University Press.

Irigaray, L. (1985). *The Speculum of the Other Woman* (G.C. Gill, Trans.). Ithaca, NY. Cornell University Press.

Jacobs, A. (2007). *On Matricide. Myth, Psychoanalysis and the Law of the Mother*. New York: Columbia University Press.

Kristeva, J. (1987). *Black Sun: Depression and Melancholia*. New York: Columbia University Press.

Linder, R.M. (1948). The Equivalents of Matricide. *Psychoanalytic Quarterly*, *17*, 453–470.

O'Brien, M. (2007). The Dialectics of Reproduction in O'Reilly, A. (Ed.). *Maternal Theory*. Ontario: Demeter Press.

Rozmarin, M. (2016). Staying Alive: Matricide and the Ethical-political Aspects of Mother-Daughter Relations. *Studies in Gender and Sexuality*, *17*(4) 242–253.

Sheehy, M. (2012). The Maternal Postmodern: Commentary on Rozmarin's "Maternal Silence". *Studies in Gender and Sexuality*, *13*(1), 24–28.

Stone, A. (2012). *Feminism, Psychoanalysis, and Maternal Subjectivity*. New York: New York.

Chapter Ten
The Case of Tina

My patient was a 60-year-old woman with grown children. She divorced her abusive and unfaithful husband when her children were 8, 10, and 12. Although he was wealthy, he paid little in child support. She went back to get a college degree and now works at a low paying nonprofit job. She still has huge student loans to pay back and currently lives with her daughter and family. Tina came into treatment because she was not getting along well at work. Her productivity was acceptable but she felt that "on bad days" it suffered. She also had numerous physical complaints including chronic fatigue, diabetes, and obesity. She lived in a tiny apartment in subsidized housing and had continuing conflict with the apartment manager as well as her boss and colleagues at work.

The first three years of treatment were very productive. She proved to be an intelligent and insightful individual who could work well in twice-weekly therapy. I believe that my primary function was to serve as a container, a "facilitating environment" if you will, in which Tina could recount and process the events of her turbulent and tragic life. She focused many of the sessions on issues at work. She was a hard worker but stayed in her cubicle in an isolated corner. She spoke very little to co-workers but felt that she was scapegoated by them and by her boss. While her work was acceptable, she was often chastised by her supervisor for circumstances for which she felt unfairly blamed.

DOI: 10.4324/9781003413677-11

Though the patient had told me about her childhood and the real horrors that she encountered, she had not felt safe to discuss them at length until later in the treatment. She described a "narrator" voice which could recount the trauma and abuses she had suffered. It was as though they had happened to someone else, not her. She described a nightmarish existence in which she lived in a tiny house with her mother and many children. Her older brother had sexually abused her, though her mother became angry at the patient when she described the situation. Her step-father had actually beaten another brother to the point that my patient thought he was going to kill him. The patient tolerated her mother's verbal and physical abuse until she was finally able to leave the home and move in with her boyfriend. She did not attend her mother's final illness or her funeral though she continued to note the anniversary of her mother's passing.

As Tina became more able to talk about these experiences she described her mother as beautiful—a cabaret singer who dressed very fashionably. Her grandmother—a tiny woman who smoked incessantly—was hated by the mother. She had no decent place to live, but her daughter, the patient's mother, never offered to help. My patient's great-great-grandmother was alive when she was a child and provided a lot of stability for everyone. She lived in an old farmhouse which the patient remembers fondly. Her great grandmother however was "not right in the head" due to an illness in early adulthood. She lived with the great-great grandmother and was in bed most of the time. At some point the great-great grandmother "fell" down the stairs and died of injuries. As details of this history emerged, it turns out that her daughter, the great grandmother, had pushed her down the stairs and this crime had been covered up in the family for decades. It was, I believe, after the patient revealed this "family secret" that our positive treatment relationship began to erode.

Initially, Tina had progressed in a number of areas. Her physical health had improved and her relationships at work had become more manageable. Her productivity increased considerably and she began to receive accolades for her accomplishments. She was able to tolerate an evaluation with her boss without the debilitating panic attacks that she had suffered previously. Our relationship was also quite positive and could be characterized as idealization on her part. Though she had insurance to cover the sessions, I had agreed to forego the co-payments. Tina frequently told me how much she appreciated my efforts on her behalf.

WHEN THE POLITICAL BECOMES PERSONAL

When, in the summer of 2016, a cast of characters appeared on the political scene, so exaggerated that no one could make them up, my patient's defenses were perforated—permeable—and all her angry badness emerged passionately in regard to the political campaign. She was a fervent Bernie fan and, though she could contribute little financially, she attended rallies, hung posters and flyers, and made her views known wherever she could. She felt that he spoke for her and others who were struggling to make ends meet as she had for much of her life. She resonated with his message of paying off student loans, making college education free, making health care accessible, and other ideas that he espoused.

At some point she began to inquire who I was going to support. I had in the past shared with her some personal information, that is, that I had grown children and that I was married. My office is in my house so that some of this data was readily available. Based on what I believed to be a comfortable relationship I felt that I could share with her that I was a Hillary supporter. I added that I had been a lifelong feminist and that I was excited to have a woman president. She seemed to be accepting of the differences in our political beliefs.

She did, however, continue to educate me about her beliefs that the DCC was favoring Hillary, that is, working in her behalf, and that the campaign was treating Bernie unfairly. When the nominating process was over, Tina was angry and embittered and believed that Hillary was nominated unfairly. When I indicated that I was still supporting Hillary, I became conflated with a powerful mother figure—rich, smart, conniving, even murderous—and certainly in her mind incapable of providing nurturing support. At this point, a dizzying confluence of factors—intrapsychic, interpersonal, and cultural—had hit like a tsunami and neither of us, my patient nor I, were able to stand. The psychic womb that we had created had been perforated. Tina acknowledged that she was angry at me and that she couldn't believe that I would support Clinton after all the information that she had given me about what she considered to be the shady goings on of the DCC. She asked me angrily how I could do this when what she had told me was true. We had only a few more sessions before I was taking a summer vacation. We scheduled a session after that time but in the meantime she e-mailed that she wanted to take a break from treatment. I have not heard from her since that time.

The abrupt ending in Tina's treatment was, I believe, a complicated mix of cultural, inter-personal and intra-psychic factors for both patient and therapist. When a powerful mother imago entered the room in the person of Hillary Clinton, it proved too much for either of us to hold. We were confronted with a present-day mythical figure—rich, smart, conniving, and motherly—who awakened within us the frightening or liberating possibility that she could rule the world.

The stakes were high for each of us but we came from vastly different perspectives. Tina's female body and her early and young adult life experiences had left her extremely vulnerable. In the first years of treatment I was able to provide a psychic womb for her but, when outside political factors entered the fray, she, once again, became permeable. Up to that point I had been a helpful emotional container for Tina. We had co-constructed a secure setting in which repair could occur. She was better able to navigate the inevitable insults and injuries that she encountered at work; manage what had been overwhelming anxiety when she had an evaluation; stand up for herself; and negotiate a more positive relationship with her daughter. Her physical health improved, as did her ability to communicate with doctors abut medical issues. She was able to channel and mitigate her rage about their inability to provide "cures".

But when the political contest began in earnest, it became a very personal battle for Tina. As a devoted Bernie fan, she became enraged when he was not nominated. She said that she would support Trump over Clinton. It was as though the figures at the center of the fray had become real characters in her life. They were archetypal to be sure—cartoon-like in their manifestation of cultural stereotypes. Bernie Sanders was the mature and benign uncle who gives out candy at Christmas time. He promised relief from student debt, free college, and the possibility of a standard of living that, in the case of Tina, could lead her out of grinding life-long poverty. His campaign gave her hope. Set against this possibility were, in the perception of many, two unappealing choices. One was a morally bankrupt man who possessed an ego structure which apparently demands continual expressions of adoration and who espoused a platform of bigotry, racism, homophobia, and misogyny. His opponent and the eventual winner of her party's nomination was a rich, smart woman who had attained a place of power, not just in the home but in the world. She was, again in the perception of many, a stereotypical feminist whose power as the leader of the free world would be enormous. Ultimately the choice was between an arrogant "alpha male" and an uppity feminist who had ground her way to the top, pushing aside any who stood in her way. Given the generations of mothers in Tina's life and the seemingly unfettered power that they held, her only alternative was a man who could somehow contain that unimaginable female force. My support of Clinton became a betrayal, an act that left her unprotected from treacherous female power.

But why had I left my stance of relatively noncommittal political neutrality? In my defense, I am quite certain that I was not alone in doing so. The political climate of 2016 had, for many, intruded into the clinical setting and into our lives. Neutrality in that setting became very challenging and possibly even unhelpful. In her commentary Blue Chevigny addresses this point, stating that discourse within sessions has changed:

> [Patients feel that] they are living in a new context since the election. They often want to talk about politics during sessions, and I have dispensed with whatever illusion of neutrality there may have been previously…The experience of learning about extraordinary developments in politics and processing them simultaneously with my patients…has been an equalizing force in the therapy room.
>
> (p.23)

She goes on to say, however, that we as therapists must not lose sight of the fact that we still possess a level of authority and that our opinions, however mildly expressed, carry significant weight. In his review of the same book, Matthew Oyer (2016) argues that psychoanalysts, given their focus on internal concepts like the unconscious, have overlooked any attention to social-cultural concerns. He states that "a theory is needed that can elucidate the mediating processes by which external oppression is internalized … the reality principle's imprint on the unconscious mind" (p.20). These concepts illuminate the notion of "the social third" as discussed by Muriel Dimen in *With Culture in Mind* (2011). She states that "individual psyches and psychoanalytic dyads are infused and delimited by discursive systems" and that "we cannot undo its powerful staging effects because they are the very stuff of which are meanings and intentions are made" (p.49).

In any case, the national scene had entered our personal lives as never before. I too found myself struggling to remain politically neutral and, in many instances, made it clear that I was not supporting Trump. Many of my patients in the liberal community where I practice were appalled that we would elect this candidate and I affirmed that conclusion. There were situations in which I found it necessary to offer a level of reassurance as well as a reality check on the accuracy of a patient's perceptions. In one instance, a woman who had been raped as a teenager, expressed real terror at the prospect of a man, one who apparently glorified sexual assault, being elected president. The conflict had also unearthed profoundly felt antagonism in our culture and the arguments had become personal. Families became divided; friendships lost as opposing factions defended their views. As an example, I follow the listserv of a group of well-known psychoanalysts and I found myself witness to an online shouting match in which name-calling and derogatory comments erupted among these dignified individuals who were discussing the current political quagmire. As an electorate we became bitterly divided, in the midst of a nasty "divorce" with incredibly intense feelings on both sides and nobody willing to compromise. Mediation efforts continue to fail and we have hurtled toward hostile rhetoric and even violence.

But what was my personal stake in this predicament? As a lifelong feminist I was thrilled with the nomination of Hillary Clinton. Here was a woman who had fought her way to the top in the face of so many obstacles. She was hard-driving and powerful but my reaction was "so what!" Men do it and women have to work even harder. I found her to be nurturing and compassionate. I knew of anecdotes in which she had comforted an aide whose dog had died as well as other acts of kindness that seemed motherly to me. She represented a powerful female, one who could provide protection from an aggressive male whom I perceived to be stalking her on national television. It appeared to me that the generations of women in my family who had railed and struggled, though largely unsuccessfully, against the male yoke were, at last, vindicated.

In the context of this therapeutic relationship I had, quite possibly, supported Hillary as my protector—*Liberty Leading the People*. Perhaps she could shield me from the barrage of anger that I knew to be "behind the scenes" with my patient. Maybe she could protect both of us from the morally bankrupt power-hungry individual who was the alternative candidate. As an incredibly toxic and intrusive campaign, it represented in many ways the age-old battle of the sexes: the "father from hell" versus the archaic mother—mystical, mysterious, and yet extraordinarily powerful over our earliest and most vulnerable selves. I do believe that I am not alone in experiencing this particular campaign as having an emotional valence that we have seldom, if ever, encountered.

The turning point in our relationship came when Tina remembered or first revealed to me that her great-grandmother had indeed murdered her own mother and that this had been a family secret that had altered the lives of ensuing generations. Had she touched too closely my own family secrets? Was I compelled to counter her attacks with a larger-than-life woman who could protect the country and, most especially, me? The archetypal mother as represented by Hillary was, for me, a protector, a champion, while for Tina, she signified a powerful but evil sorceress who embodied the traits of the generations of mothers from whom she had to escape. The good mother/bad mother was in full display.

In hindsight, I realized that the pressure toward enactment was enormous. I had known that at some point I would become the "bad" mother just as I had initially become the "good" mother. As a good, even idolized figure, I was able to provide the support that Tina needed to make significant gains—a safe environment, a mirroring of her feelings, the attunement which had been absent in her early life. But when I had revealed my hand as a Hillary supporter, quite possibly because I needed protection from Tina's rage and murderous impulses, I then became conflated with the all-powerful evil mother—dangerous, exploitive, and even deadly. The convergence of inner and outer influences, combined with my patient's rediscovery of her great-grandmother who had murdered her own mother created a vortex of guilt, shame and anger that became too much for either of us to bear.

The "mother myth", as illustrated in the case of Tina, still prevails within our culture. That myth may still have held sway in the US presidential election of 2020, given our collective perception that female candidates are "not electable". "Mother" remains a powerful figure, the repository of our hopes and dreams for a better life and, nearly simultaneously, the cesspool from which all of human evil eventually emerges. From this perspective, we dare not contemplate her real experience, her pain in childbirth, her sorrow in war, her fear for her children or the unending pain and tedium of rearing them. So she remains, sequestered in our individual and cultural unconscious and unchanged through eons of time. As Jacqueline Rose states, "motherhood is…the place in our culture where we lodge or rather bury, the reality of our own conflicts, of what it means to be fully human" (2018, p.I). Yet mothers, if they could be allowed to speak freely and openly, would have much to say about the ills that plague our society. It is more than past the time when we must free them from the entrapment of their mythical status and enable them to address us from the core of humanity that they represent.

References

Chevigny, B. (2017). Politics in the Therapy Room. *Dimension/Review: A Quarterly Psychoanalytic Forum, 16.*
Dimen, M. (Ed.). (2011). *With Culture in Mind*. New York: Routledge.
Rose, J. (2018). *Mothers: An Essay on Love and Cruelty*. New York: Farrar, Straus.

Chapter Eleven
If the Ego is a Body Ego...

We get the God part. She is Charity, Benevolence, Liberty Leading the People, and a host of other esteemed virtues. She is Mother Russia; one of the great ocean liners which often bear female names; and, though absent in Judeo-Christian thought, the role model for dozens of female deities.

But where does the quite human mother stand? She bleeds on a monthly basis when the discarded uterine lining is expelled. She may or may not experience debilitating cramps, depression, or mood changes which have historically rendered her unclean and even, currently, make her unfit to accomplish much of anything at "her time of the month".

Let's say that her pregnancy is wanted. Has she gone through fertility treatments, IVF, or other modern conveniences that allow her to have a baby? Does she feel unspoken guilt and shame, as did my beloved aunt who was barren well before the present fertility treatments? Does her partner want a child? Is the partner committed to help care for the baby, at least financially? Is she required to have a male child, which was certainly the case throughout much of our history? Has she already lost a child? What is her living situation? Will there be enough baby formula for the baby (a real concern in the spring of 2022)?

If the pregnancy is unwanted, will she be able to make her own decisions or will the government (male) make decisions for her? Will she be

DOI: 10.4324/9781003413677-12

reduced to the status of an endangered animal species whose every offspring is protected by higher (than the mother) authorities?

If she carries the baby to term will the labor be difficult or easy? Will she need a C-section or other modifications to help her deliver? Will she have help to care for her infant? Will she carry the baby in a backpack so she can continue working the rice fields? How will the infant be accepted by her partner or other siblings? Will she get ANY time off?

These are immediate practical concerns. The physical changes in the mother's body, as with any physical modification, will also be felt psychically. What of the plasticity of the fecund body? How does one experience the feeling of gaining 60 pounds in nine months? Or the awareness of a growing belly, all out of proportion with one's ordinary stature? What about the discomfort in later stages when organs are being shifted about to make room for the growing fetus; pressure on the bladder; clumsy movements accompanied by comparisons to a baby whale? What does the mother do with these changes? Does she imagine herself as a monster? Is she proud of her burgeoning belly? I did have moments of pride and dreamt, in fact, that my uterus was on my face. It was as if I was finally able to acknowledge that I was a sexual being. I enjoyed walking through the U of M campus where I was in my doctoral program and seeing the sophisticated university students averting their eyes at the sight of a pregnant woman.

Another issue for the mother is that of permeable boundaries. She is carrying a little stranger, and, whether welcome or not, it is a breaching of boundaries. She and the fetus are in one body. Her body is responsible for the nutrients, the oxygen, and the very life of the baby. Mother and baby are merged. How does mother negotiate the separate life of the infant or the youngster or the grown child? She has a relationship with the being that begins inside her body and is replicated nowhere else. It is a consideration for the baby as well but that has been documented. The mother's physical connection with her child is played out psychically and must be understood. I hypothesize that it is related to the greater frequency of "borderline" conditions in women than in men.

The issue of boundaries does not end with the birth of the baby. Mother and baby are closely linked in the first few months of life. The health and well-being of the baby are totally dependent on the mother and it is her job to keep the baby alive. If she is breast-feeding, the breast itself is, as it has been for centuries, the essential food source. In the most primitive of terms, the baby is literally "eating" the mother. What is that experience like *for the mother*? What is it like to possess life-giving breasts which are, at the same time, the highly sexualized focus of male attention? How does she process the knowledge that her breasts are both a food source and a sexual symbol?

Breast-feeding itself can be frustrating and painful. What if a baby wants to eat every two hours around the clock? What if the mother cannot produce enough milk? What if the baby bites her? What if the breasts become infected? Perhaps most sinful and secret are the pleasurable and sensual sensations that the mother feels. The mutual gaze of mother and child can be intense and powerfully sweet for both, but it is almost forbidden to speak of it. Are those experiences, like the memories of giving birth, dissociated? Too painful or too precious to contemplate or share? They are "normal" and "essential" but I believe they are so far beyond ordinary physical experiences that they are in themselves traumatic and thus dissociated.

Chapter Twelve
Maternal Grief/Maternal Madness

Can we place these two topics—grief and madness—together? As clinicians we are aware that unresolved and unacknowledged grief can appear as madness. I recall a client who came into my office because she was hearing the sounds of a baby crying—not her real babies. She also had an image of a man pinned to her ceiling above her bed—older; no one she recognized. She was neatly and attractively dressed and oriented fully. She said that she had a total of five children—three from previous relationships of both her husband and herself. She became pregnant and learned she was carrying triplets. Her husband was appalled and insisted that she abort one of the babies. She did so but very reluctantly.

It was after the births that she experienced what might be termed a postpartum psychosis. Though I only saw her for two sessions, her experience seemed to be encapsulated and thus was not affecting her otherwise adequate functioning. In the time we had, we discussed the possibility that she was angry at her husband for insisting on the abortion. Her guilt about the aborted fetus was undoubtedly at play in the experience of the crying phantom baby, as well as the unknown man pinned to the ceiling. She was also seemingly at odds with her husband who was not supportive of her pregnancy.

 DOI: 10.4324/9781003413677-13

Another client who sought treatment was barely able to care for her infant. She had been working full time at a demanding job and was suddenly at home—isolated with no family nearby. She had not been going out at all. Her husband was travelling for work. She was virtually immobilized. We discussed the need for her to seek support in the form of paid childcare and to venture out with friends. We discussed the idea that she did not have to be with her baby all the time but, in fact, needed breaks to care for herself.

My mother's loss of the baby Elizabeth colored her life and those of my sister and me. My sister was born soon after the loss of the infant. I was born 4 and a half years later when my mother was almost 41. Somehow I became the "dead baby"—not exactly a replacement child but dead in a most basic sense. I learned to be very still; not to feel or, at least, not be aware of feelings other than acute separation anxiety. I studied ballet and there I was free to move about in the stylized dances of the ballerina. But at my core, if you will, I felt dead. My skilled analyst was at last able to make that interpretation so that I could begin my journey back to life.

I don't believe my mother ever recovered from the loss of Elizabeth. She went through a deep and untreated depression at menopause. She exacted her own version of "perfection" from her daughters, perfection that could only be achieved by her lost and angelic daughter. Her soul became twisted in a manner that contained her grief but left her tears unshed. It was a grief that she was instructed not to feel since she was told that she "could have other children". It was as if her lost baby was one of a dozen kittens that could easily be interchanged.

Andre Green has stated that the idea of "normal maternal madness" is neither shocking nor surprising.

> It is sufficient to reflect for a moment on pregnancy and maternity with sufficient perspective and objectivity to grasp that throughout this period, for the woman living through this experience, there is a complete remodeling of her feelings in relation to the world, and the organization of her perceptions which are entirely centered on the infant [NOT]. The mother's sensitivity to the most imperceptible signals take on a quasi-hallucinatory quality for onlookers. Pregnancy and maternity take on a miraculous dimension for the mother; they satisfy wishes of omnipotence and the wish to be, for the infant, all that

> he is for her, this unique incomparable object to whom all is owed and all is sacrificed. It is when this madness does not appear that we have reason to suspect that the matter is disturbing".
>
> (p.245)

Green further states that "the mother must contain the infant's instinctual life" (p.246). The mother also (p.244) "remodels her feelings in relation to the world and the organization of her perceptions which are entirely centered on the infant". In what Green terms "normal maternal madness", the woman must "accept and contain her own instincts" and function as "an auxiliary ego, a container and a mirror for the infant" (p.245). His description is, in my view, a state of being that has the potential to overwhelm the maternal ego in ways that may never be repaired or reinstated. It is a drastic type of change that undoubtedly affects the mother, for good or ill, and for the rest of her life.

In *Mothers: An essay on love and cruelty*, Jacqueline Rose further links maternal grief and madness. With great sorrow and compassion, she illuminates the ways in which mothers are blamed for all that is wrong with the world. Mother carries the grief, the cruelty, the marginalization, and the silence, and it is driving her mad. She speaks at length about Elana Ferrante, who has coined the term *frantumaglia* which describes the sensation of being torn apart, "a miscellaneous crowd of things in her head, debris in a muddy water of the brain" (pp. 168–169). It is a way of expressing a feeling for which no language exists, that is, "language not as a tool but in the form of words that endlessly slide from our grasp" (p.169). As Ferrante describes, it is "a hum growing louder and a vortex-like fracturing of material living and dead: a swarm of bees approaching the motionless treetops" (p.170). From the perspective of Jaqueline Rose, then, every mother carries grief; cruelty; and the badness of the world; and from this she is to make joy, engagement, protection, from a world gone mad. How then would this not drive her insane?

Toni Morrison brings full circle the impact of the world's unrelenting cruelty on mothers. Her novel *Beloved* talks about the effects of slavery on a family and particularly motherhood. If a mother does not "own" either her baby or herself, it makes loss and separation even more intense. The book describes Seth's murder of her yet unnamed baby and her explanation of it to Denver, to Paul D., and the baby, Beloved, who comes to haunt their home.

Under normal circumstances, a woman who kills her baby is generally regarded as "mad". But Seth is responding to the horrors of slavery and she cannot bear for her child to suffer in that way. Her own subjectivity had been experienced between her escape to freedom and the murder of her baby to preserve that freedom. Seth loves her children. Morrison writes:

> The best thing she was, was her children. Whites might dirty her all right, but not her best thing, her beautiful, magical best thing—the part of her that was clean. No undreamable dreams about whether the headless, footless torso hanging in the tree … was her husband or Paul A; whether the bubbling-hot girls in the colored-school set by patriots included her daughter; whether a gang of whites invaded her daughter's private parts, soiled her daughter's thighs and threw her out of the wagon. She might have to work the slaughterhouse yard but not her daughter.
>
> (p.196)

At the end of the novel she is allowed her subjectivity. Paul D. helps her to grasp it for a moment. She says, "Me? Me?" She questions the hierarchy of motherhood over selfhood. The novel both explains and challenges that hierarchy. It allows her to recognize Beloved as her child and to begin to recognize herself.

For good or ill, mother stands at the portals of life and death. It too frequently drives them mad and countless mothers know this. But we, all of us, dare not to look into the chasm.

References

Bronte, C. (2006). *Jane Eyre*. New York: Penguin Classics.

Green, A. (2018). *On Private Madness*. New York: Routledge.

Morrison, T. (1987). *Beloved*. New York: Vintage Books.

Rose, J. (2018). *Mothers: An Essay on Love and Cruelty*. New York: Farrar, Straus, and Giroux.

Chapter Thirteen
Time Out of Mind
Dissociation in the Virtual World

While greatly facilitating ease of interaction across time and geographic boundaries, the virtual world presents an unreal environment comprised of instant connection and gratification. Online encounters are employed as seemingly fulfilling alternatives to "live person" relationships. Our culture has enthusiastically embraced this surrogate reality in the form of online journals, chat rooms, and gaming as well as internet pornography and sexual solicitation. It has become a significant part of modern society and will undoubtedly continue to do so as new generations find ever-innovative ways to integrate it into daily life.

Yet we are already aware that excessive preoccupation with the virtual world may prove disruptive both to productive functioning and the development of satisfying relationships. Phrases such as "internet addiction" have already entered the lexicon and refer to behaviors that are similar to addictions to drugs and alcohol, resulting in academic, social, and occupational impairment. Whether we, as psychoanalytic clinicians, are technophiles or troglodytes, it is almost certain that excessive preoccupation with virtual reality will enter our consulting rooms along with our patients. As such, we must regard it as a significant aspect of mental functioning and then focus the powerful tools at our disposal in our attempt to understand it for ourselves and our patients.

DOI: 10.4324/9781003413677-14

An individual's over-involvement with the internet can, however, prove difficult to engage in the clinical setting. It may become sequestered, outside of time, intensely private, couched in shame, and underreported. It thus remains a personal space, the repository of dissociated thoughts and emotions, unlinked to the self-reflexive ebb and flow of feelings that foster awareness and change (Aron, 2000).

In addressing this new and puzzling phenomenon I will first briefly summarize the data on internet abuse. I will then examine the concept of dissociation and apply it as a way of understanding those forays into the virtual world as time out of mind—experiences that are disconnected from thoughts and feelings that would assimilate them into an ongoing biographical narrative. Finally, I will present two clinical vignettes that illustrate the variety of forms that internet abuse may take. I will make the case that each of these illustrations, one involving a young boy and the other a women in her mid-thirties, represent a manifestation of dissociative defenses. Though their use of the internet is outwardly very different, it is similar in its function as a split-off and alien interpersonal world that provides protection for a fragile self state. I will discuss the need to invite the dissociated material into the therapeutic dyad so that it may become a conscious and integrated aspect of the self. I will examine the therapeutic process as one involving both verbal interpretation and relational grounding in the person of the therapist.

A VIRTUAL TSUNAMI

Since the 1990s the internet has become a defining characteristic of our society, flooding cultures with revolutionary technology that has altered dramatically the way we do business, access information, maintain contact, and relate as human beings. A wave of technological advance that grows and changes almost daily, it is a vital part of the lives of young people who grew up in its wake even as older generations struggle to learn and keep up. It has opened a new universe of communication and worldwide contact and its effects upon our culture are only beginning to be addressed. The positive consequences are easy and obvious while the negative aspects remain subtle and insidious. It places, as never before, the control of a very powerful tool in the hands of an individual. The social impact of the virtual world is and will undoubtedly continue to be far-reaching. For the psychoanalytic clinician its force will be felt as it affects the individual, both in his or her psychological functioning and in the authenticity of relationships that he or she is able to achieve. We might well ask whether or not our interface with the virtual world has the potential to change what it means to be human.

Phenomena such as MySpace (TIME, 2006) or Second Life allow users to create whole new people with different careers, social status, age and gender. Second Life mimics real life in every way ("Second Life", 2006). Users meet other people, throw parties, attend church, and even open businesses where they sell virtual goods. Some users begin by treating it as a game but quickly realize that it is real. Some say it has changed their lives by allowing them to create a whole new identity or overcome social anxiety. Its dark side involves those who spend 40 to 100 hours per week at their computers or hide their excessive involvement from others.

Social networking sites such as MySpace have become extremely popular ways for teenagers to meet and interact. As documented in the news, security issues have become a nightmare as in the well-publicized case of the 16-year-old girl who secretly flew to the Middle East to marry a man she met there. While the site has protective measures in place, such as prohibitions against posting last names, street addresses, and phone numbers, it is difficult to check the accuracy of required data such as name, gender, and date of birth.

In somc instances it appears that users are attaching to the virtual world as if it were a "real" relationship. In fact, it has many of the dimensions of human interaction. It can occur in real time. People may reveal private thoughts and feelings in ways that allow them to become better acquainted. They work, play, fight enemies, initiate romance, and accomplish a multitude of other activities in interactive ever-changing modes that closely approximate real life.

In *Extra Life: coming of Age in Cyberspace* (1998), David Bennehum tells the story of his childhood experience with computers and describes his belief that emotional bonds are now related to technology. As an adolescent he had a self-described addiction to video games that he compares to an addiction to heroin. He expresses the feeling of comfort that he derived from playing old computer games like Donkey Kong, much as one might receive comfort from seeing one's childhood home.

In some circles, interaction in the virtual world passes as a viable and even superior manner of human relating (Inter Change Transcript on Virtual Communities. http://www-personal.umich.edu~wbutler/IC12695PI.html). An online discussion about the strengths and weaknesses of virtual communities indicates that some respondents believe that a more open and honest type of communication can develop online than in real life. While participants note the absence of face to face interaction, that particular drawback is outweighed by the possibility of talking to a variety of people from all over the world.

Many of the respondents in the virtual discussion viewed as a strength the opportunity to play a different role than one does in real life. Instant prejudices based on physical characteristics do not exist. The computer network breaks down barriers of time and space and allows us to bring together a large pool of minds to share information, experience, and knowledge. While in real life individuals hesitate to communicate their true opinions, it is easier to do so online because they don't ever have to meet the people they are talking with.

Some participants cite as an advantage the lack of physicality, allowing us to concentrate more on our words and what we are really trying to say than on how we say it. The leader of the discussion, Wayne Butler (2007), asks whether indeed face to face interaction is the best way to build human relationships. He raises the question as to why the warm and emotional face to face contact is also the mode in which people clam up and become less than genuine. He concludes that we should go with the more "honest" mode that is available in virtual communities.

Some respondents however mourned the loss of face to face interaction, noting that participants seem uncomfortable talking to real people after conversing freely with strangers online. They pose the question as to whether we will lose the ability to communicate in physical ways. Others state that it may "cheapen" the culture by diminishing genuine human contact. The opinions of those who are less enthusiastic about online communication coincide with authors such as Winnicott (1974), Eigen (1993), and Beebe (2005) who consider face to face contact to be central in the development of deep mutual attachment between mother and infant and indeed throughout life.

Excessive internet use has been called an addiction by authors such as O'Reilly (1996) and Young and Rodgers (1998). Recent reports have indicated that some online users are becoming addicted to the internet in the same way that others have become addicted to drugs or gambling. Such compulsive overuse has been linked to academic failure, reduced work performance, and marital discord. A study by Young (1996) has endeavored to develop a workable set of criteria that could be effective in diagnosing addictive internet use. Gambling addiction was viewed as most akin to pathological internet use since it is an impulse-control disorder that does not involve a substance or intoxicant.

Young employed questions such as the following to distinguish normal from dependent internet users: Have you repeatedly made unsuccessful efforts to control, cut back, or stop internet use? Have you lied to family members, therapists, or others to conceal the extent of involvement with the internet? Dependent users spent a mean of 38.5 hours per week "surfing the Web" in activities other than academic or employment-related purposes while normal users spent an average of 4.9 hours per week. Thus dependent users were spending nearly eight times the number of hours per week as normal users. Chat rooms and multi-user dungeons (MUDS) were the media most frequently accessed by dependents.

Other researchers such as Grohol (1999, 2005) and King (1999) have however questioned the concept of addiction as an accurate description of internet overuse. Grohol points out that the there are people who read too much, work too much, or watch too much TV. Yet we do not refer to their behavior as addictive. Grohol points out that many of the exploratory surveys have methodological weakness and theoretical inconsistencies. While they may describe a behavior they are not able to ascertain the cause in any compelling manner. In his article "Is the Internet Addictive or Are Addicts Using the Internet?" King points out that research has frequently failed to address the nature of previously existing mental illnesses such as anxiety, depression, or relationship issues.

INTERNET USE AND THE DEVELOPMENT OF THE SELF

The question of whether or not the internet is addictive is beyond the scope of this paper. From a psychoanalytic perspective it may be used, as Monder (2007) has pointed out, in a variety of ways, including forays into alternative experiences and lifestyles that facilitate beneficial changes in self perception and ways of being. It is when the individual user is either unwilling or unable to integrate that vast array of information into his or her own real existence that it may become problematic. When it becomes a substitute interpersonal world, controlled by the click of a mouse and outside the demands of time, genuine emotion, and meaningful engagement, it has the potential to draw us away from the essential characteristics of social interaction, a 21st century manifestation of social alienation and anomie.

A humorous and graphic example of that kind of involvement comes to mind from the TV show *South Park*, in which the participants become so engrossed that the real world, including the demands of the body, has no meaning. A group of children have vowed to rescue the father of one of the boys by slaughtering his enemies in a virtual game. In order to achieve their goal they must sit in front of the computer for days on end. One of the boys even persuades his mother to bring food to the gaming area and, eventually, a chamber pot, so that he can take care of his bodily needs. In this extreme example, the virtual world has become paramount, and reality, an insignificant distraction.

At first glance the internet in its various manifestations may appear to present an unprecedented opportunity to create experiences that simulate one's fantasies and play them out with an endless supply of enthusiastic participants or vengeful opponents. It has an astonishing capacity to create an interpersonal world that is *almost* real and it presents the user with tantalizing and even seductive choices and experiences. One can be anyone, anywhere and at anytime. A person has unlimited access to an infinite array of opportunities to fulfill every fantasy, grant every wish, or satisfy every desire. They can face any fear or conquer any enemy, all at the click of a mouse. It provides a form of entertainment that we have never known before and are unlikely to give up. If we leave it at that—an unprecedented and fascinating diversion as well as a unique way to access information and connect with people worldwide—we can appreciate its power and potential longevity. But as a satisfying and fulfilling manifestation of meaningful interpersonal experience and an avenue for healthy psychological development, it possesses subtle but important deficiencies.

We know that across the centuries human beings have found a myriad of ways to create rich and varied fantasy worlds. The embodiment of imagination is present in all the art forms: drama, literature, music, dance, and the visual arts, beginning with the paintings found on the walls of ancient cave-dwellers. Such expression in any form allows us to project our inner world in a way that permits others to perceive it and resonate with it as some approximation of their own experience. Isn't that what the internet is all about—a venue that allows millions of users to engage with each other within an ever-changing dream world? I would suggest that the answer is both yes and no. While it permits the user to interface with an infinite variety of imaginative expression, it forecloses, for reasons that are not entirely clear, the crucial interchange between fantasy and reality.

When the world of fantasy in any form becomes a seductive alternative that breaks with ongoing experience, it disrupts the biographical narrative that is critical to the development of agency and the functioning of the relational self. It is no longer part of the vital and continuing perception and processing that moves freely between observation and experience even as the individual operates both intellectually and emotionally. A number of theorists have discussed this function and its impairment in those who have suffered early trauma.

Ogden (1990) would portray such an adaptation as an impairment in symbolic thinking, a concretization of fantasy such that it loses the "as if" quality. He might describe it as a dissociation of fantasy and reality, a state in which one no longer informs the other. The individual has the potential to become lost in fantasy in a way that destroys its possibility for modifying and enlarging reality. The mind loses its capacity to move freely among affective and intellectual elements. In Ogden's view, those individuals that are particularly susceptible to this kind of impairment have suffered early trauma such that they have failed to give personal meaning to experiences that have been too terrible to feel.

When the world of fantasy becomes a seductive alternative that breaks with ongoing experience, it disrupts the biographical narrative that is vital to the development of agency and the functioning of the relational self. It embodies a loss of what Aron (2000) calls self-reflexivity or the reflexive function of the mind. In Aron's terminology, self-reflexivity involves the capability of moving back and forth between observation and experience while being able to function both intellectually and emotionally. It is an essential self-function that allows the integration of mind and body, thought and affect, observation and experience, and, in my opinion, is an aspect of mental operation that is particularly vulnerable to excessive internet involvement.

As Fonagy and Target (1995) point out, in the presence of unbearable trauma, the psychic contents split, cordoning off the intolerable affect or memory. The person is able to go on even while suffering a reduction in awareness of surroundings, thus becoming numb or detached. He or she is no longer able to construct a continuous biographical narrative, one that moves comfortably and freely within the mind and has the ability to access feeling, fantasy, and memory, as it relates to the interpersonal world of the present.

Under such circumstances one's ability to act from a cohesive sense of agency is not destroyed but "repackaged" in unlinked states of mind (Bromberg, 1994). Impairment in symbolic thinking occurs so that reality and fantasy are experienced as parallel but disconnected phenomena. Relationships are possible but highly regulated and lacking in spontaneity. Adaptations may take place that require a modification of self-structure in the form of guilt, shame, and low self-esteem so that the individual takes on responsibility for wrongs committed by others. Intimate needs remain alive but sequestered, carefully insulated and ready for danger, so that trauma can never again arrive unanticipated.

TIME OUT OF MIND

The virtual world with its myriad of personae and infinite variety of props, settings, and storylines appears, in fact, tailor-made for someone who, although able to function, does so by means of dissociative defenses. The DSMIV-TR defines dissociation as a break in the normally integrated functions of consciousness, memory, identity, or perception of the environment (American Psychiatric Association, 2000). The Psychodynamic Diagnostic Manual (PDM Task Force, 2006) understands dissociative disorders as a diminution or lack of the ability to synthesize information from their various senses (sight, sound, smell, touch) into an integrated experience of what is happening to them. Complex social experiences and their associated affective states cannot be taken for granted, but may be split off or perceived as alien. Wilkinson (2005) addresses the multiplicity of definitions of the phenomenon and suggests that it reflects the complexity of what analysts may experience as they work with patients who dissociate. Fonagy and Target (1995) also note the complexity of psychological states one may encounter in working with dissociative disorders.

For the purposes of this discussion I would like to stress the view of dissociation expressed by Shore (2001), Siegel (2003), and others as a disruption in the development of agency or self, that is, a relational, intersubjective self that has emerged from the earliest and most fundamental experiences of relating. When that early experience supports the infant in the management of physiologic and affective states, minimizes unsettling ruptures, and provides an option for the reparability of inevitable failures, he or she is able to construct a more or less continuous biographical narrative. In the absence of secure human relatedness (Bromberg, 1994) and a stable, though largely nonverbal and unconscious, foundation for internal affect-regulation, the individual splits off intolerable feeling states, giving up an experience of wholeness in order to go on. The ability to act from a cohesive sense of agency is not destroyed but re-packaged in unlinked states as "time out of mind".

Unable to hold in conscious thought the intolerable and conflicting feelings of love and hate, guilt and reparation, the person functions by splitting off unmet needs or unmanageable affect, defining it as "out there", a part of the not-me experience. The individual may be able to maintain contact with reality but does so by severely distorting a sense of self, agency, and relationships with others. In Klein ian terms (Envy and Gratitude, 1980), he or she occupies the paranoid-schizoid position in which projected parts of the self can be managed by controlling another person or another action figure in a video game. Aggressive impulses are assigned to someone else. The individual becomes the object of projected persecution and feels justified in seeking revenge for injustices. It becomes a narcissistic adjustment in which the normal give-and-take of relationships is minimized or, shall we say, deleted.

The therapeutic task requires that patient and therapist co-construct a transitional reality within which faith in the reliability of human relatedness can be restored. It requires interpersonal engagement that combines affective honesty and safety. The goal is to provide a foundation of reparability that allows for successful negotiation of interpersonal transactions that are essential to the re-building of trust. We may explore the destructive or addictive behavior but we also seek to disengage it from the underlying self-state which has had to be preserved in the interests of psychic survival (Davies and Frawley, 1994; Bromberg, 1995). In the absence of reliable care-giving, the individual has learned to substitute dissociative defenses such as excessive involvement in the virtual world as a way of regulating helplessness, desire, and the relative unpredictability of human contact. The therapeutic aim is to search for the relational bind embedded in the computer use, formulate it as a conflict in symbolic terms, and explore it within the new relationship developed in the transference (Director, 2005).

Such a task is not easily accomplished. The behavior may remain heavily guarded in a conscious way so as to protect vulnerable self-states. Once it is addressed it must be recognized as a psychic achievement, a coping mechanism that has assured that parts of the self can go on in spite of unbearable trauma. As treatment progresses the patient may reveal an inner life dominated by a never-ending war between parts of the self, that is, internal voices, sadistic and unrelenting, that the patient needs to still by giving each one some of what it wants but never satisfying all (Bromberg, 1994). One may encounter separate centers of attention that communicate with and control the total personality. Though they may not be so extreme as to be called a dissociative identity disorder, they may be distinct in their views of reality and in their inability to communicate with each other.

The undoing of frozen and sequestered self states entails recognition both of the coping mechanisms that have protected them, however destructive they may be in the present, and, ultimately, a re-visiting of the trauma that brought them into being. When trauma has been experienced in the context of earliest relationships, its processing is very much limited to the right brain, given that the left brain capacity for verbal memory and processing is not yet fully developed. Verbal and symbolic interpretation will be insufficient then to capture and re-define those basic experiences (Beebe, 2005; Wilkinson, 2005). The analyst must recognize the presence of the terrified child within the functioning adult and address communication in ways that will reach both.

TIMMY—THE BOY WHO LIVED IN TOONTOWN

Timmy is an angel-faced boy of ten who was caught in the middle of a custody battle between his parents who had separated when he was one and a half and divorced when he was four. Initially the parenting arrangement had been amicable. The parents had lived close enough that Timmy was able to spend part of the day with each parent. When the father remarried and moved farther away, the daily schedule became much more difficult to maintain, particularly since the mother was unwilling to do any of the driving. Alternating weeks with each parent made public schooling problematic. When I saw Timmy, he was being home-schooled by his mother. His father objected to this arrangement however, because he felt that his son spent too much time playing on the computer and lacked social contact with other children. He was suing for full custody so that his son could live with him during the week and attend the public schools.

The choices for Timmy were bleak. When he was with his mother he did indeed spend a great deal of time playing on the computer. A weekly schedule of home-schooling activities as provided by his mother indicated the following:

> August 28th: A few hours on the Toontown website.
>
> August 29th: Corrected spelling on Toontown site and added additional toon tips; Timmy created a back button in his gif animator. Text was not displaying properly. Suspect syntax error but could not find it. Toontown with Sarah in the evening.
>
> August 30th: Toontown with Sarah in the morning.
>
> August 31st: Toontown with Sarah in the evening.
>
> September 1st: Toontown with Nathan; Timmy read to me for half an hour from Toontown's maintenance and update logs. He has a tendency to substitute similar-looking words for each other, but he understands what

> he reads and is interested in the history and development of the game. Read more of *Mansions of the Gods* while Timmy was playing Toontown and waiting for his father to come. Timmy's comment: "Whenever anyone says they see dragons in a book and they take someone else to see them, the dragons are always gone".

In addition to grave emotional problems Timmy's mother has been diagnosed with serious immune-related disorders. She has been in chronic pain and finds it difficult to keep up with the demands of work and housework. When Timmy was small she acknowledged that her housekeeping was unacceptable. At the time of the evaluation she kept the home rigidly immaculate. She is a writer and writes literary erotica, including rape fantasies and descriptions of actual rapes, though she assured me that Timmy has his own computer and does not have access to this material. Her mother has a Ph.D. in computer engineering and both her mother and brother write video games. For these reasons she stated that she felt comfortable with the amount of time that her son spends playing on the computer.

Timmy's father is a maintenance engineer and at the time of the evaluation was living with his second wife and her two children, a son who is eleven years old and a daughter who is nine years old. The son has a mild but observable physical handicap and the daughter has been diagnosed as bipolar. When I observed Timmy with his father and step-family, the parents described the difficulty of the daily transitions and the problem of integrating Timmy into the ongoing schedule of homework, chores, and bedtime routine. They stated that when Timmy first arrives at their home he is "hyper and crazy". He plays with his step-sister and they amplify each other's energy levels. His older step-brother views Timmy as something of a rival and emphasized that, in spite of his limitation, he could swim more laps than Timmy. During the family interview Timmy appeared very quiet and said nothing unless asked a direct question. This was in contrast to his animated behavior with his mother and, eventually as he became more comfortable, with me.

In my evaluation of Timmy I would describe him as mystified both by his own feelings and the emotions of those around him. He acknowledged to me that he gets "hyper", more so at his dad's house than his mom's. He said that he doesn't say a lot at his dad's house and that it is hard to think of much to say when everyone is talking. He feels a "whole bunch of anger" inside sometimes but he is not allowed to express it to either parent. He gets mad at his mom when she wakes up crabby in the morning and gets tense about something small that he has done. He gets upset with his father when his father makes him do a lot of chores. He is aware that his parents are fighting about him and he is puzzled by it. "Why can't they stop fighting and work it out so everybody's happy?" he says. I asked him if he felt sad when his parents fought. He replied that he didn't but that he usually just stayed away to give them "their space".

Timmy also related that he spends a lot of time being bored and lonely. He gets bored at his father's house when everyone but him is doing something else and he is not allowed to play computer games. He finds public school boring because they do the same things over and over and he doesn't have time to spend on his own creative projects. His computer world provides the stimulation he is seeking but even there he can feel unhappy and lonely. He feels sad when he loses a fight on a video game and knows that he will have to "fight all over again". Even on Toontown people seem to hate him. He tries to put it out of his mind but then he remembers it again.

As part of the evaluation I asked Timmy to draw a self-portrait. He drew a roomful of toys and computer games—including a game cube and controller, a bucket of Legos, and his computer. He showed it to me and then said, "I forgot to draw myself". It was as if his own person had become lost in a world of cartoons and computer games, an escape from the real world in which he is constantly disrupted and moving between two very different households. Though his parents appear to be interested in his welfare, they are, in fact, more interested in their ongoing controversy than in their child. He finds them too often preoccupied with other things: his mother with the computer and his father with "hanging out" with his present wife.

Toontown provides a refuge for Timmy: a safe place where he can act out angry feelings and exercise control over what happens to him. It is a multi-player online game that lets you "live the life of a Toon". You can create your own character, build an estate, play games with friends, and explore amazing places. It is advertised as "always growing, always changing, and as wild as your imagination". But we learn that there are evil forces at work in the form of Cogs—evil robot business types who have arrived to take over the town. Cogs can't take a joke so the one way to defeat them is to crack them up with an arsenal of gags—seltzer bottles, cream pies in the face, anything that makes them laugh. Each player earns laugh points by completing certain tasks. The more laugh points, the stronger your Toon will become.

Need friends? It's easy. Simply click on the Toon you would like to make friends with and a message will pop up telling you if that person is interested in being your friend. Is your Toon sad? No problem. Fill up your "laff" meter with more gags and your Toon will be happy again. It's a cartoon world where friends appear at the click of a mouse and evil Cogs are defeated in Punchline Place, Loopy Lane, or Silly Street.

Toontown sounds harmless enough and even entertaining. It provides an alternative from the extremely violent video games in which the primary task is to hunt down enemies with an ever-increasing array of brutal weaponry. As an occasional distraction and outlet for imaginative play it seems ideal. But Timmy is not engaging with it in that way. For him it has become an alternate world—a safe space in which he can exercise a measure of control away from the chaos and unpredictability of his real life. He can make friends and defeat enemies, gain power by filling up his "laff" meter, and it provides some measure of stimulation and engagement that he is unable to experience with his parents and family.

CASEY AND THE HOUSE PEOPLE

Casey is a single professional woman in her mid-thirties whose work involves apprehending internet sexual predators. She came into treatment feeling that she was under-performing at work and socially isolated. She wanted to be in a long-term relationship with a man and eventually marry and have a family. She had to force herself to go out and meet men and she didn't understand why.

Early in treatment Casey expressed unremitting anger toward her mother from whom she is partially estranged. She described her mother as a self-centered woman who was seldom able to focus on her daughter's feelings without making her aware of what a burden she was. The father left their family when the patient was two years old and after that her mother dated a number of men. Casey recalls instances in which the mother would bring men home and engage in sexual activity so that the patient could hear them from a nearby bedroom. The mother married two more times, the second husband being an alcoholic. She is currently living with her third husband.

Casey portrays her father as a child-like man who married too young and was unprepared to be a parent. She visited her father sporadically throughout her childhood but does not regard him as a father figure.

She has memories of waiting for him by the window and then having him not show up. He didn't pay child support on a regular basis so her mother was compelled to support the children on her own as best she could. Casey also has an older sister who is married with two children. She has a half-sister who is her mother's child and a half-brother who is her father's child. Her half-brother is also married with two children. The patient maintains close relationships with all of her siblings.

In many ways Casey presents as an ideal patient. She appears cooperative and cordial and is intelligent, psychological-minded, and insightful. Though moderately overweight she is attractive and well-groomed. She pays her bill on time, seldom cancels, and consistently greets me pleasantly at the beginning and end of each session. She began treatment with once weekly sessions and quickly agreed to meet twice weekly. She has been on the couch at three times a week for about three years. Her productions are colorful, humorous, and sometimes brilliant but progress has been slow. She will characteristically assent to an interpretation but then meticulously dissect every word of it. She has actually asked for a dictionary to check on the specific meaning of words. If one is not available she tells me that she goes home to look up a word if she is not exactly certain of its meaning. My response has been to allow her the absolute freedom to explore every nuance of every word and to resist the impulse to force an interpretation on her. I consider her careful reactions to be a protection of an extremely vulnerable self state of which we have been able to catch only brief glimpses.

In an atmosphere in which her autonomy has been acknowledged and respected, the patient has come to know that her verbal productions and outer air of congeniality are only a small part of her total being. Over time she has introduced me to a whole internal cast of characters whom we have named the "house people". There is the "housekeeper" who is the administrator and most closely aligned with the patient, the "me that is me". There is the "pathetic one", whining and complaining and barely able to get anything done. There is the "smart aleck", a domineering, aggressive and somewhat sadistic character who constantly berates the pathetic one. There is a little girl who sits quietly and says nothing but watches. Later we have learned of a little boy who hides behind the couch and is bad and angry. This motley crew maintained an ongoing conversation/argument in Casey's head in a way that tortured her. The smart aleck continually nagged the pathetic one. The housekeeper tried to maintain order. The little girl watched, seemingly stunned into silence, and the little boy, who only occasionally made an appearance, disrupted the whole proceeding. When Casey was at work or with people she could keep the conversations at bay. But when she was alone they dominated her life. In fact she had to be alone some portion of the time to satisfy them and let them out. They could communicate with each other but not directly with her and not with me. So she could not be with other people and in their presence at the same time.

Casey and I have spent many sessions discussing reports of the house people. Though she cannot speak with them directly she can tell me what they are saying and what they want. As we have listened to their conflicting demands with understanding and patience she has been able to redefine them as three-dimensional beings with complex needs that are intertwined with one another. The smart aleck has become more understanding of the excuses of the pathetic one and she, in turn, has been able to stand up for herself and explain her reasoning. Through that process the patient has become more accepting of her limitations and not so harshly critical of her failings.

She has in fact begun dating again, meeting men through an online dating service. This is after a hiatus of many years in which she had few, if any, dates and fended off efforts of friends and family to "fix her up". Yet dating itself has proved problematic. We have come to realize that she reacts in a nearly phobic manner when she is anticipating the prospect of meeting someone new. We have explored her responses in terms of her fears of men seeing her as overweight. The prospect of spending long periods of time in intimate contact with a man also appears frightening, both because of the physical closeness and the psychological openness it would require. Yet these explanations do not appear sufficient to explain the extreme nature of her reactions at the prospect of being with a man.

In her professional life Casey is required to review hundreds of pages of pornographic material written by sexual predators who are attempting to solicit sexual contact online. These men are apprehended when law officers posing as teenagers agree to meet them. In order to prosecute offenders the state must prove that the internet material is designed to solicit an actual meeting with the victim and that the perpetrator believed that the victim was under age but wanted to meet him or her anyway. The material is often incredibly graphic such that, during a trial, the prosecutor may warn a jury of its salacious nature in order to prepare them. The offenders can be well-known and respected members of the community or the lowest dregs of society, but they are typically in denial and unrepentant as to the harm they may be inflicting on their victims. Casey took great satisfaction in helping gather material that would implicate those she believes to be guilty, but expressed only appropriate and professionally modulated "outrage" at the heinous acts which they had committed or were attempting to commit.

It became apparent however that her associations would frequently travel from a potential meeting with a new online acquaintance to her indignation at the behavior of an accused sexual predator. In the same session she might express her carefully regulated disgust at the conduct of a perpetrator and then, her anxiety, which she fully acknowledged, at the possibility of a date with a new acquaintance. This pattern appeared often enough that we began to explore the connections. The question of whether the patient had herself been sexually abused came to the fore. The impact of her father's abandonment of her and her family became relevant. She had never acknowledged its effect, assuming that, since she had been "too young to remember", it hadn't been important in her life.

While these questions have yet to be answered it remains clear that her involvement with online predators and perpetrators of sexual solicitation is more than a professional activity for Casey. It is a world populated with males who commit monstrous acts and exploit children for their own purposes and without regrets. In that world Casey can express justifiable and regulated outrage and can act out her anger in a way that brings the perpetrators to justice and punishment. She may even meet these individuals face to face along with their families, as well as the victims and their families. She is invariably able to maintain her composure though she expresses her disgust privately to me.

Although she is under-utilizing her capabilities, Casey is functioning successfully in her professional life. She works in a difficult profession and acknowledges that it can be stressful but she is proud of her ability to tolerate the challenging material that she encounters. Indeed, when we were talking about the "house people" Casey described her professional self as living outside the house and being dismissive, even scornful, of those inside. Yet it is within her professional world that she has sequestered her most intense and irretrievable feelings of rage, revulsion, hurt and exploitation. Here she can keep them neatly packaged, carefully regulated and, most importantly, far away from her personal relationships with men, her mother, her father and anyone who has the power to hurt her.

In a recent session Casey expressed the following:

> Well, okay. I was reading 30 pages of blog. There were e-mails from a perpetrator to a cop posing as a 13-year-old girl. I felt nausea. Like not in your mouth. But it was

nausea. I couldn't continue. I was crying. But I had to do it. He said, "Masturbate and rub your fingers in it. Then rub it on paper and draw a heart around it and send it to me". I've read worse. I've been disgusted. But it was not at the deep visceral level.

I asked why now?

I don't know. I am meeting a date tonight. Maybe I am anxious about that and don't have the energy to hold the feelings down.

I said that the feelings seem to be connected, at least in time.

She said that she was not aware of it. She said, "Ellen, I don't like having feelings. It's upsetting".

At the next session she said that she didn't have much to say. She had nothing to say about the date. I said, "Follow your thoughts. They may be in disguise".

She said that she couldn't get to them. "It's like a table with things on it that I can't reach". I asked what might be on the table. She said that it might be a pepper shaker or a newspaper. I asked her what made it so she couldn't reach them. She answered that it was like fog but not exactly. It was "swarmy", like a swarm of gnats. "It's like a swarm that you bat away. It's a swarm. It's a psychological phenomenon. Swarm is no longer a word. Swarm. Swarm. It has lost its meaning. It's like when you say a word over and over and it is just a bunch of letters with no meaning".

Coincidentally in his book *Nausea* (1969) the great existentialist philosopher Jean-Paul Sarte describes a similar experience in response to his observation of a man molesting a young boy in a park. In his discussion of Sartre, Toronto (1999) states that the hero of the book, Antoine, is totally cut off from society. He lives alone, speaks to no one, and neither gives nor receives from anyone. His deprivation is such that he has lost the ability to give meaning to events. Sartre describes his protagonist as "a teller of tales … surrounded by his stories and the stories of others … he sees everything that happens to him through them and he tries to live his life as if he were telling a story" (1969, p.39).

Before long Sartre's hero, Antoine, not only lacks the ability to relate stories and events but also loses the ability to label simple objects and ideas in a meaningful way. He recounts several nauseating experiences in which objects—including a doorknob, a beer glass, and trees—lose their definition. He can't describe what they really are because he realizes that "we have so much difficulty imagining nothingness … things are entirely what they appear to be—and behind them there is nothing" (1969, p.96). He also observes that "the words had vanished and with them the significance of things, their method of use and, the feeble points of reference which men have traced on their surface" (p.127). Ultimately Antoine experiences these realizations both as freedom and, simultaneously, as a kind of death. All reasons for living have been extinguished. He poignantly describes a kind of psychological abyss, a terrifying space without attachments or connections that might constrain and at the same time support his existence.

This literary example comes to mind because it seems quite possible that Casey, in the course of her treatment, has also come to the edge of her own psychological abyss and has, indeed, peeked over its perimeter. It is no surprise that once she has done so she would recoil in horror and return to the safety of her considerable intellectual defenses. There she can live in relative security among the house people and thus avoid encounters with the emptiness around that highly restricted internal environment.

But fortunately Casey seems to possess a quality that Sartre's hero does not and that is a desire to "go on being". She retains a measure of hope based on some positive attachments in her early life, and, quite possibly, in the connection and grounding that she has experienced in her relationship with me. She is tempted to turn and run but she does not. She is committed to her treatment and understands, intellectually at least, that painful emotions lurk in and around the "nothingness". In a recent session, for example, she described having a massage to alleviate the knotted muscles in her neck. Toward the end of the massage session she felt something release and everything turned "pink". She got out as fast as she could because she felt that she was going to cry.

In recent weeks reported external events have conspired to make Casey's work undeniably personal. In the session following a session that was cancelled for the July 4th holiday, the patient reported that it has been a "terrible" few days. A male in-law of her closest friend was about to be arrested on a charge of participating in internet child pornography. At first the patient was struggling with the ethical issue of whether or not she should warn her friend that the arrest was about to take place. Then she began to describe her reaction at work and when she was on the phone with her friend. She had cried hard on both occasions and was surprised that she had reacted so intensely. She was quietly shedding tears as she talked about it with me, an extremely rare occurrence in the years that I have been treating her.

She then said that her work had finally become personal. She could see and feel the tragic impact on the victims and the families of both victims and perpetrators. She said that it was like she had been working in a slaughter house, slaughtering cattle. She had been able to do her work by remaining comfortably detached. Then without warning one of the cows looked up at her before she slit its throat and she had to run out screaming. We puzzled about whether her feelings about her work had been there all the time or whether they were situational, only in response to the arrest of her friend's in-law.

One might imagine that Casey's reaction to these recent events and the ties to her own past would now become obvious, a slam-dunk. But that has not been the case. She has neither recollection nor reason to believe that she was sexually abused as a child. We are still in the early stages of exploring the impact that her father's abandonment has had on her. She is well aware that her mother's self-centered preoccupations have had a devastating effect but has only begun to touch the hurt that has resulted from that relationship. At a conscious level she acknowledges me as a benign facilitator in her quest but I am still only beginning to be allowed to communicate with the people who inhabit her inner world. We continue, slowly and patiently, to untangle those threads that are connected to emotional "hot spots" that alert us to a bubbling cauldron surrounding the unbearable pain she has experienced.

DISCUSSION

Let us now consider the very different examples of internet use provided by Timmy and Casey. Timmy is a child who under the guise of home-schooling spends many unsupervised hours in an interactive world of cartoon figures, one in which he can make things happen, influence the story line, and manipulate characters in amazing ways that have never been possible before now. Casey is a productive adult who uses the internet to accomplish work-related goals in a manner that most of us would find laudable. Yet for both of these individuals their use of the internet has become a repository of thoughts, feelings, and encounters that are disconnected from their real life experience. Infinitely repeatable, the internet encounters are immune to the self-reflexive capabilities that would allow them to be accessible to memory, emotion, and fantasy and thus integrated into an ongoing biographical narrative.

According to the home schooling logs provided by Timmy's mother is it likely to assume that he is spending 30–35 hours on the Internet. By definition (Young, 1996), this amount of involvement would constitute an addiction. His mother writes internet erotica. His grandmother and uncle design video games. Without some major intervention it is likely that this will be Timmy's life. His father appears to be attempting to extricate his son from this world but provides a stressful and chaotic alternative that would only magnify the anxiety of this already fearful young boy. The fighting between his parents is unrelenting and Timmy finds his only solace in the illusory world of Toontown. There he can express anger, fight bad guys, make friends, and have a sense of agency that is so lacking in his real life.

In many ways Timmy is fighting for his psychic existence. In the drawing of his room he forgets to draw himself. Like the imaginary dragons one encounters in a book, when someone tries to prove his reality he disappears. His parents profess to care for him but their commitment to their ongoing battle too often takes precedence over Timmy's welfare. For him the internet is a survival tool. He can "live" there and until someone is able to acknowledge and contain his fear, his anger, his fragility, and his longing he will most likely continue to do so.

But as Ainslie (2007) states, this adaptation is, at best, marginal. She questions as to whether the anxiety Timmy experiences at his father's house stems from a confrontation with real and unpredictable human interaction that threatens his omnipotent and grandiose self, a self that he can more easily maintain on the internet. Does that mean that his self-representation is an assemblage of computer parts and games? Do computer games serve as a transitional object for Timmy? Or, more ominously, do they function as a soothing primary attachment, a "cyborg-mother"? Ainslie warns that, while Toontown may be a reliable, predictable place, it is not real in any way that would allow this young boy to accommodate his "finely textured" human needs.

For Casey, the use of the internet is a much more circumscribed part of her life and as such could easily go unnoticed as a barrier to healthy functioning. It was not mentioned as a presenting problem. It is certainly justifiable as part of her work and it is not something she does in her leisure time. Yet over time it has become clear that her investment with it serves to bind aggression, fear, revulsion, and powerlessness. It perpetuates her view of men in general as untrustworthy predators in ways that permit no modification from real life encounters. It is a fixed part of her experience to which she reacts with only measured professional disgust. It also allows her to maintain appropriate distance from the as yet undetermined experiences of her own life which were too horrific too contemplate.

This carefully contained experience with internet predators and her participation in seeing that justice is done has allowed Casey to master again and again her fear and powerlessness in relation to men. One might consider it a successful adaptation were it not for her relative social isolation and conflicted anguish about dating. Rather, her use of the internet represents an escape hatch, very much like an addiction of any kind, in which unacceptable feelings and memories are sequestered outside of time and inaccessible to healthy modification and integration. While recognizing its necessity as an escape mechanism, we have begun to disentangle and support the vulnerable and fragmented self state that it protects.

In the process the barriers around this circumscribed piece of her life have begun to crack. In the session noted above she was able to express the nausea she felt as she read 30 pages of pornographic blog. Instead of the articulate and carefully worded associations we have also begun to have periods of "nothing", lapses into silence that Casey calls "unintentional". Another time shortly after the "nausea" session she again described the experience of having a word lose its meaning after having said it a number of times. I understand this to be a kind of detachment from the reality that words impose and, quite possibly, a retreat to the mind and experience of the silent little girl who remains yet to be engaged.

As Ainslie (2007) points out, it is the little girl who most closely parallels what Casey does on the internet, that is, a silent observer, much as she was in relation to her mother's sexual activity. She has retreated from the toxic relationship with her mother into a defensive attempt at mastery, proud of her ability to tolerate the material she must read every day. Like Sartre, that 20th century chronicler of social alienation, she disassembles the noxious material and drains it of meaning so that she can hold it. But, as does Sartre, Casey pays a heavy price in terms of her relationships to the object world and her relatively schizoid existence.

So it will continue to be a struggle for Casey and I to remain engaged when we are both convinced that boredom and detachment are greatly to be preferred to the intensity and unpredictability of genuine emotion. We will spend time on treacherous paths where the road is "swarmy" and covered in fog, where emotions are pink and unintentional silences abound. With luck and perseverance we will find our way to those experiences in which Casey's life broke down and the hurt became too horrible to bear alone.

In conclusion, I believe it is safe to say that the internet and the virtual world it presents have changed our lives forever. It has and will continue to be a significant part of our culture and a defining aspect of human interaction. As with any other change of this magnitude its effects will be both positive and negative. Its positive impact is phenomenal, with the capability to connect and integrate the human family in ways that we have never dreamed possible. It can, however, become a substitute world, controlled by the click of a mouse and outside the demands of real time, genuine emotion, and meaningful engagement. To that extent it has the potential to draw us away from the essential characteristics of human development, a 21st century equivalent of social alienation. It is at this juncture that psychoanalysis, with its wealth of understanding of individual and interpersonal functioning, can make a significant contribution, placing the engagement with the virtual world in an appropriate perspective and reminding us yet again of the amazing and timeless capabilities of mind and imagination.

References

Ainslie, G. (2007). Time out of Mind: Psychoanalytic Explorations of Patients' Excessive Engagement with Virtual Reality. Paper presented at the Spring Meeting of the Division of Psychoanalysis (39) of the APA in April 2007.

Ann Arbor News. (2006, November 6). Second Life, E1 and E2.

Aron, L. (2000). Self-Reflexivity and the Therapeutic Action of Psychoanalysis. *Psychoanalytic Psychology, 17*, 667–689.

Beebe, B. (2005). Faces-in-relation: Forms of Intersubjectivity in an Adult Treatment of Early Trauma. In B. Beebe (Ed.). et al. *Forms of Intersubjectivity in Infant Research and Adult Treatment* (pp. 1–45). New York: Other Press.

Bromberg, P. (1994). "Speak! That I May See You". Some Reflections on Dissociation, Reality and Psychoanalytic Listening. *Psychoanalytic Dialogues, 4*(4), 517–547.

Bromberg, P.M. (1995). Psychoanalysis, Dissociation and Personality Organization: Reflections on Peter Goldberg's Essay. *Psychoanalytic Dialogues, 5*(3), 511–528.

Butler, W. (2007). Inter-change Transcript on Virtual Communities. Retrieved from http://www-personal.umich.edu~wbutler/IC12695PI.html.

Davies, J.M. and Frawley, M.G. (1994). *Treating the Adult Survivor of Childhood Sexual Abuse.* New York: Basic Books.

Director, L. (2005). Encounters with Omnipotence in the Psychoanalysis of Substance Users. *Psychoanalytic Dialogues, 15*(4), 567–586.

Eigen, M. (1993). *The Electrified Tightrope.* Northvale, New Jersey: Jason Aronson.

Fonagy, P. and Target, M. (1995). Dissociation and Trauma. *Current Opinion in Psychiatry, 8*(3), 161–166.

Grohol, J. (1999). Too much time online: internet addiction or healthy social interaction?. Retrieved from http://www.research.net.

Klein, M. (1980). *Envy and Gratitude.* London: The Hogarth Press.

Ogden, T. (1990). *The Matrix of the Mind: Object Relations and the Psychoanalytic Dialogue.* Northvale, New Jersey: Jason Aronson Inc.

O'Reilly, M. (1996, 15 June). Internet Addiction: A New Disorder Enters the Medical Lexicon. *Can Med Assoc J., 154*(12), 1882–1883.

Sartre, J. (1949). *Nausea.* New York: Penguin Books.

Shore, A.N. (2001). Minds in the Making: Attachment. The self-organizing brain, and developmentally-oriented psychoanalytic psychotherapy. *British Journal of Psychotherapy, 17*(3), 299–328.

Siegel, D.J. (2003). An Interpersonal Neurobiology of Psychotherapy. In M.F. Solomon and D.J. Siegel (Eds.), *Healing Trauma.* New York: Norton.

TIME (2006, July 3). My Space, pp.35–36.

Toontown. (n.d.) http://play.toontown.com/playersguide/printchapter.php?printsection=1

Toronto, D. (1999). *To Define Freedom.* Unpublished Manuscript.

Wilkinson, M. (2005). Undoing dissociation: Affective Neuroscience: A Contemporary Jungian Clinical Perspective. *Journal of Analytic Psychology, 50,* 483–501.

Winnicott, D. (1974). *The Mirror Role of the Mother and Family in Child Development: Playing and Reality.* England: Penguin.

Young, K. (1996). Internet Addiction: The Emergence of a New Clinical Disorder. *Cyber Psychology and Behavior, 1*(3), 237–244.

Young, K. and Rodgers, R.C. (1998). Internet Addiction: Personality Traits Associated with its Development. Paper presented at the *69th annual meeting of the Eastern Psychological Association in April 1998.*

Chapter Fourteen
Maternal Trauma

The case for maternal trauma has been made again and again. Mother has, indeed, a tsunami of forces that render her experiences both as trauma and as dissociation. Jacqueline Rose (2018) has skillfully outlined the array of forces that inflict cruelty upon mothers even as they attempt to love their offspring. It is this array, this deluge, inflicted upon mothers throughout history that has, of necessity, rendered their experiences dissociative.

In this discussion I have focused on those cultural, religious, theoretical, and biological imperatives that have created over millennia an experience for mothers that is unsustainable in conscious thought. As with Freud and the Oedipus story, I have chosen the Clytemnestra myth to illustrate the cruelty that has been inflicted on mothers—rape, the murder of her children before her eyes, the blatant infidelity of her husband, and, last but not least, the condemnation of the gods.

The Old Testament as a purveyor of culture has provided a narrative that references mothers as "wombs"—essential to the continuation of the patriarchal line but without acknowledgement as subjective beings. The anonymity of women throughout history has been documented in *Anonymous is a Woman* (2020) and reinforces the idea that if one does not exist, one cannot have a story.

DOI: 10.4324/9781003413677-15

The 19th century quilters, those stalwart "sunbonnets" who tamed and populated the American West, provide a window into the private lives of women and mothers. They were not the sheriffs, the gunslingers, or the cattle barons whose heroic tales are known and admired. They told their tales in their art—the beautiful quilts that provided both warmth and the companionship of fellow quilters. They represented their sorrows, their joys, and their accomplishments nonverbally, as is often the only venue available to mothers.

The gods of psychoanalysis, both traditional and relational, have continued the trend, either ignoring or vilifying mothers as the origin of lifelong developmental wounds. Mother becomes either an insignificant entity or a mysterious nonverbal miasma from which a child must escape to enter the patriarchal world of language and logic. Rosemary Balsam has taken a huge step forward in her focus on the female maternal body. She confronts our verbal and patriarchal theories as she points out the absence of attention to the amazing experiences of pregnancy. She alerts us to the idea that women's essential organs are largely invisible—a mystery to all and sundry even now.

To this list of affronts we may add the very fact that subjective experience is mostly articulated verbally and in the context of an ongoing conversation with another verbal person. We no longer subscribe (or at least I don't) to the idea of a one-person universe. We create our self states in relationships with significant others. But when mothers are mothering an infant or small child that "other" is non-verbal. Mother must, of necessity, communicate nonverbally so that her corresponding subjective experience is not recorded in language. The experience is stored as sensual, body-based, and inaccessible to the conscious mind. It is a breeding ground for dissociation.

The topic has been taken up recently by Gemma Hartley (2018) as it describes the cost of "emotional labor". It is mentally and emotionally exhausting and consumes every aspect of a mother's life. Hartley notes the obvious, that it is unpaid labor and yet requires that mothers see to the comfort of everyone around them. She also observes that psychoanalysis tells us that caregiving is invisible just as women are. She urges women to communicate about the burdens of emotional labor and the need for men to share equitably in that role. I fear, however, that communication alone will not shift the balance. The roots of the problem are entrenched in patriarchy and, as Gilligan and Snyder point out, the attendant fears of ongoing caring and loss.

References

Ansary, N. (2020a). *Anonymous is a Woman*. Revela Press.
Ansary, N. (2020b). *Woman: A Global Chronicle of Gender Inequality*. Los Angeles, CA: Revela Press.
Balsam, R. (2012). *Women's Bodies in Psychoanalysis*. New York: Routledge.
Gilligan, C and Snider, N. (2018). *Why Does Patriarchy Persist?* Cambridge, UK: Polity Press.
Hartley, G. (2018). *Fed Up.: Emotional Labor, Women, and the Way Forward*. New York: Harper One.
Rose, J. (2018). *Mothers: An Essay on Love and Cruelty*. New York: Farrar, Straus, and Giroux.

Chapter Fifteen
The Dissociated Maternal Self

Berthe Mason was sequestered, hidden away. Someone else had to stop the wedding in order to note that Rochester was still married. She was at best an embarrassment (screaming and dithering and all that sort of thing) and, at worst, a nothing, a nonentity whose usefulness no longer existed. Now, however, in retrospect, I realize that she personifies a dissociated self state, a figure in the attic, one that, like a trauma state, appears at inopportune times.

Green's description of mother's state of mind sounds like madness to me. Her identity must become "shapeless" or "liquid". It is an apt description but not necessarily one to be consciously desired.

Green states that the mother lives with the infant in an "autistic" state, a "universal sensory-dominated mode of experience" (p.30). She must be capable of immersing herself in the infant's sensory world as "she allows herself to de-integrate into relative shapelessness … she allows her identity as a person and as a mother to 'become liquid' in a way that parallels the internal state of the infant" (p.202). It involves "a dialectical tension between the shapelessness and the formed, the primitive and the mature, the mysterious and the familiar" (p.198). This frame of mind is in addition to the baking of pies, the PTA, arranging for lessons and the like which Odgen unfortunately considers a brittle and schizoid approach to mothering. Both skills are required—one an ability to

DOI: 10.4324/9781003413677-16

respond to the nonverbal cues of the infant as well as the growing child and the other, a set of highly evolved organizational skills, currently requisite in the socialization of children.

The inner life of the mother is destabilized by cultural tropes that have a long and seemingly revered history. Rose states that "having nothing of her own to grapple with—being all for her child at the cost of her own inner life—is the very definition, or at least the unspoken agenda, of being a mother" (2018, p.193). Andre Green (2018) has, early on, alerted us to the idea of "normal maternal madness", given the changes required of the mother as she "looses [sic]" herself in order to focus on the child. He speaks of the semi-hallucinatory quality of the communication between mother and infant and the wonder that an observer might experience as he watches the amazing synchronicity that occurs.

It is a song without words but it happens because the mother is able to access her own nonverbal world. In my view, it easily falls into the realm of the "unformulated self"; Stern; the "primitive edge" of experience (Ogden); and yes, the "psychotic core" (Green).

Rose asks the reader what would happen if we listened to mothers; if we could translate their experience linguistically. What if we didn't assume that mother's "primary maternal occupation" is easy or even possible? What if we addressed the messiness of the human body *of both baby and mother*, or the erotic charge the mother feels while breastfeeding? What if we acknowledged in linguistic (public) terms the central role that mothers play in the preservation of the species and preserved their presence as persons of importance rather than their mere depictions on funeral urns? What if we allowed the mother an existence for herself? Significant and potentially traumatic aspects of maternal life are not communicated to others or acknowledged by the mother herself. That is the very essence of dissociation.

References

Green, A. (2018). *On Private Madness*. New York: Routledge.

Ogden, T. (1989). *The Primitive Edge of Experience*. North Vale New Jersey: Jason Aronson.

Rose, J. (2018). *Mothers: An essay on love and cruelty*. New York: Farrar, Straus, and Giroux.

Stern, D. (2003). *Unformulated Experience*. New York: Psychology Press.

Chapter Sixteen
Mother
An Eternal Enigma

What is the cost to the human race if mother remains an enigma? I have endeavored to show in this volume that she has been so from forever. The epic tales that delineate our culture to this day have shown her to be the object of cruelty, of obeisance, and of oblivion—a womb that perpetuates the species but whose subjectivity has been universally disregarded. She possesses huge responsibility without authority—the acknowledged most difficult position in any organizational structure. She is, of course, unpaid and yet her work requires the most sophisticated of human responses. If she is a biological mother she undergoes a birthing experience which in earlier days might have led to her death. I have often pondered the thought that I could have died in giving birth by Caesarian section with my fourth child.

Her mind is an enigma even to herself for many reasons. When our culture, developed as it has over millennia of time, fails to articulate our history, our heroism, our joys, our bereavements, we lose a significant way of defining who we are and who we can become. Mothers have few role models within the pages of history and yet our duties determine all life as we know it. We are left, often, alone to figure out what will keep our babies alive; how we will get them enough food to eat; what will make them decent citizens; who will drive them to their ballet lessons. We protect them from the insanity of the world even though we have

 DOI: 10.4324/9781003413677-17

little say in the decisions that perpetuate it. In war-torn areas we shelter our children even though the wars are seldom of our making.

I am reminded of the scene in *Gone With the Wind* when Rhett Butler tells Scarlet that he is going back to join the fight. She begs him not to leave her but he insists that she is selfish because she does not want him to fight. Meanwhile, she is left driving a carriage in the pouring rain while in the back the very ill Melanie is trying to keep her newborn baby dry. Scarlet has no food and will find none when she reaches the burned out wreckage of her beloved Tara. She is far from selfish, but her duties merit little consideration when compared to the bravery that war requires.

The maternal body has also been an enigma until Balsam called it to our attention. The reproductive organs are internal—a mystery in ancient times and to this day. Babies were once thought to appear as a homunculus, that is, a fully formed tiny human inserted by the father and expelled by the mother. Freud has stated that the ego is a body ego but the maternal body is never addressed in his theory.

The time in a woman's life in which she bares and raises children is such that it interrupts her own development. It requires her to focus on her child and any attempts to pursue other interests are considered selfish. The over-arching altruism that is deemed necessary is apparent in no other human relationship. Early infant research has outlined a type of engagement and attunement that is, quite simply, not possible, on an ongoing basis, especially given the other responsibilities that mothers typically have.

Childcare is lonely. The years spent in rearing children are not with a verbal partner but with a being who is, initially at least, nonverbal. There is no affirming linguistic scaffolding that reciprocates our thinking. We are told again and again that we form our personalities in relationships. But a baby is nonverbal. Mother cannot have a verbal connection with the infant. The linguistic interchange is not present. We have called this experience semiotic or the "REAL"—somehow unknowable and thus worthy to be obliterated, such that mother, in the view of some theorists, must be "killed".

The collective culture insists that a baby returns our care and love by her charming squirms and giggles; her cries and coos; her physical excitement at our return. That is certainly true and it is one of the benefits of childcare. The cries and coos are, however, interspersed with the wails and cries that tear holes in our souls. Only scant reference is given to the fatigue that accompanies mothering. It is an exhaustion that seemingly never ends. Sleep itself is interrupted. Would these circumstances be tolerable if mothers were paid? Would it be better if people talked about it? Wrote about it? Made movies about it? Well, of course it would. Pain and suffering are always more easily endured when they are shared.

Childcare is boring. Mothers say, "If only I could talk to an adult for a little while". Engaging with a small child means that a woman must somehow return to her time with her own mother, a time of sensual bonding and synchronization of communication that may or may not have occurred in her childhood. She, in essence, must regress to an earlier state while still maintaining the adult self that she has developed. How then does she continue to grow during this period? Who does she become? I know that my own mother struggled to maintain an identity. Her self-state was fragile and my sister and I became supports, cathected narcissistically in a way that preserved her "mother" identity. We were, in many ways, her belongings. When we were good we fortified that self-state and when we were not we became the object of her rage and her paranoia. In those early days when similar feelings were awakened in me, I cringed in horror at the pain and fear that it caused in my children.

A woman's development is interrupted in so many ways. It is not only her professional life that can go offline but her self-care, her housework, her time to contemplate, or even complete a task that she has started. The constant needs, the questions, the disruptions challenge her ability to focus or make a plan. The world may become a chaotic mix of her child's emotions that she must closely monitor; the voices in her head of her inadequacy not only as a mother but as a human being; and her sense of failure in meeting a child's *never-ending* needs. As her children grow older she becomes responsible for their performance and behavior in school. As laundry strung out on the line is observed and judged by neighbors, her offspring are observed by pastors, teachers, friends, and family as to whether or not they are clean, well-fed, mannerly, and productive.

Reference

Gone With the Wind. (1939). Movie by MGM Studios: Hollywood, CA.

Chapter Seventeen
Resolutions

The experience of mothering means that a significant portion of her life exists outside of awareness. She may understand her role as child bearer and care giver but her private world, the day-by-day joys and sorrows; the miscarriages and still-born births; the sacrifice of her own initiatives; the crazy-making demands of children, small and large—demands that no one could meet—are not available to her conscious mind. They exist beyond words and, if they render her insane, she must be relegated to the attic. She becomes the "mad women" who resides there, the "attic" of her mind and ours as well.

What would be the outcome if mothers emerged from their dissociated state? What would be the effect on culture as we know it? On children? On mothers themselves? Jacqueline Rose has opined that mothers hold the cruelty of the world and that it is theirs to make it better. But what if everyone felt the savagery of war, of poverty, of oppression, of illness and death? What if we understood that the nightmares of children, held weeping in the arms of their mothers, were the nightmares that all of us must hold?

As psychoanalysts we know, of course, that it is not only the external reality that creates the terror. It is also our own fantasies, merged in ever darkening circles, that create the horrors of our inner world. But it is our mother's job to hold them, to make room for them in the mix of

DOI: 10.4324/9781003413677-18

her own terrors, real and unreal. She cannot fail in her task so she relegates her own fears to the recesses of her mind to be dealt with later or somaticized as the years go by. But what if she were allowed to express herself as a person in ways that did not involve her child and that were not deemed neurotic? What if my mother-in-law who was raising three infants in war-torn Prague in the Second World War had been allowed to express her terror? What if her needs had taken precedence over the affairs of her missionary husband who was in the business of converting people to Christianity?

We have learned much over the decades of careful and painstaking infant research about the needs of children and the elements that constitute the best and healthiest of childcare. We can describe "good-enough" mothering and we can even see the faces of the mothers as they engage or fail to engage with their infants. But research describes only the smallest part of the task. It fails to account for the context in which it occurs. Childcare does not take place in a lab. It cannot be represented in an hour of observation of one mother with her child. It does not answer questions such as the following: Is it in a peaceful home with two parents who are relatively well off? Is it in a rice paddy with a mother who carries her newborn in a sling, as Adrienne Rich so poignantly describes? Are there many children? Is there a partner who is engaged with the family? Is the partner working two jobs to make ends meet? Is it a single mother who is working to support her children? At the moment I can think of no research design that would be complex enough to identify best mothering practices in any of these circumstances.

If we collectively ignore the subjective world of mother and if, as a consequence, she does so as well, we set up an interesting dynamic, one that sets the stage for the narcissism that is so rampant in our world. We know that at around the age of eight months infants begin to realize that there is another mind, another being, with whom they must interact. Infant research has shown us that the infant strives mightily to connect with that being and that the mother may or may not reciprocate. She is, however, required to respond only in regard to her infant. That is, she is not to express "real" emotion and if she does, it is considered a flaw and, certainly, a need for guilt. The child must find only "himself" in the mind of mother. Her own lived experience is out of bounds.

The child continues on his way with the assumption that there is a being who is concerned only with "him" and that he does not have to take into account another person who has thoughts, feelings, and needs that have nothing to do with him. That assumption is played out again and again on the world stage and has done so since time began. Societal norms of every type are based on the belief that "mother" exists as a womb, essential for propagation of the species but for little else. The tender care that she provides is taken for granted and, in some modern theories, must be "killed" so that the "real" work of the world, centered in power, acquisition, and aggression, can prevail.

Yet somehow we know that mother represents the last bastion of human care and love—the prototype for all loving relationships to come. She is the portal of life, but also, alas, of death. She must hold the losses that affect the human family—the wars, the plagues, the famines, as well as the infants that pass through her being on their way to life. For those who do not make it, she carries the memories of lives that might have been. Her story is real—filled with joy but also laden with the fear and sorrow that the world has to offer. For our collective and enduring sanity, we must create a space in which she can find her true voice and we must be prepared to listen.

References

Rich, A. (1976). *Of Woman Born*. New York: W.W. Norton and Company
Rose, J. (2018). *Mothers: An Essay on Love and Cruelty*. New York: Farrar, Straus, and Giroux.

Index

A

B

C

I

J

K

L

M

S

T

U

V

W

www.ingramcontent.com/pod-product-compliance
Ingram Content Group UK Ltd.
Pitfield, Milton Keynes, MK11 3LW, UK
UKHW021307260926
475702UK00048B/792
* 9 7 8 1 0 3 2 5 3 7 9 5 5 *